FIT AT 4

FIT AT 40

Dr Rishma Dhillon Pai

RANDOM HOUSE INDIA

Published by Random House India in 2013
1

Random House Publishers India Private Limited
Windsor IT Park, 7th Floor
Tower-B, A-1, Sector-125
Noida 201301, UP

Random House Group Limited
20 Vauxhall Bridge Road
London SW1V 2SA
United Kingdom

978 81 8400 353 6

Typeset in Sabon by R. Ajith Kumar

Printed and bound in India by Replika Press Private Limited

To the two people who've helped shape my life

My husband Dr Hrishikesh Pai
and
My sister Poonam Dhillon

Contents

Foreword

I AM A 39-YEAR-OLD WOMAN. As a teenager, or even in my 20s, this isn't something I would have said out loud. But looking back at everything I have experienced so far, my voice doesn't falter. We have to embrace everything about ourselves—the good, the bad, and the ugly—to be called women in the true sense of the word. That is why I am excited about turning 40 and the life that awaits me on the other side.

I am confident of navigating my 40s well because I have taken good care of my body so far. As you all know, I had gained a considerable amount of weight post-delivery that took its time to shift. I took the healthy way back to being slim under the guidance of my gynaecologist, dietician, and of course, my gym trainer.

Even though you are confident that you are the best judge of your health, you always need a good doctor by your side. And who's more important to any woman other than her gynaecologist? They are there with you through your youth, childbearing years, and till much later in life. A gynaecologist becomes a friend with whom you can share your deepest secrets and insecurities. Someone with whom you can discuss even those embarrassing things you can't talk to with anyone else.

I wish Dr Rishma Dhillon Pai all the very best for this wonderful book she has written. It is simple, easy to read, and extremely informative. There is really very little literature and place in media given to women in their 40s, and I am glad she has brought this important phase of our lives into focus.

This book is your go-to guide to the 40s. It's going to be on my night stand for the next few years. Here's to entering the best decade of our lives.

Raveena Tandon

Meet Our Panel of Experts

EACH OF THE BELOW MENTIONED EXPERTS have contributed a chapter to my book. Thank you for taking out time from your busy schedules to help us better understand the importance of exercise, how simple changes in our diet goes a long way, and how we can reverse back the clock after we cross 40.

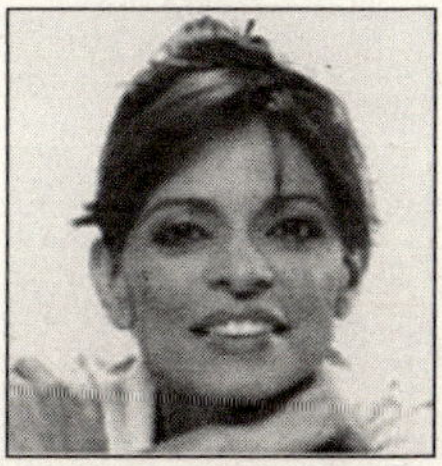

LEENA MOGRE
Fitness expert, nutritionist, and director at Leena Mogre's Fitness

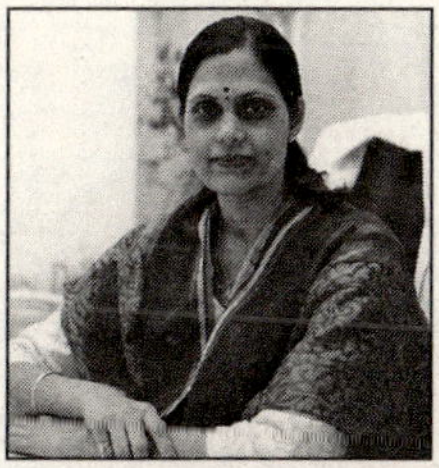

DR SARITA DAVARE
Pain and weight management consultant

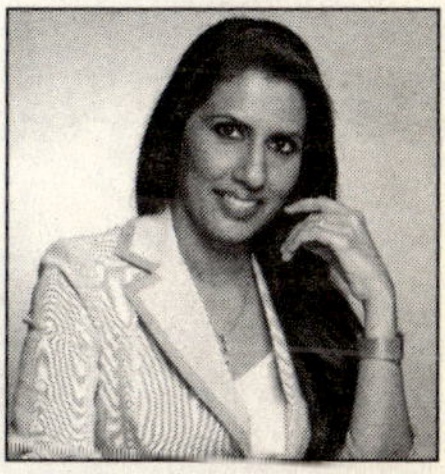

DR PURNIMA MHATRE
Chairperson, MD, Gorgeous Skin Pvt. Ltd.

Introduction

'I LIKED TURNING 40. One thing that sucks though is that your face kind of goes, and your body's not quite working the same. But you earned it. You earned that, things falling apart!'

I wish I was philosophical enough to write this. But even though these are Brad Pitt's words—a man's words—they hit the nail on the head as far as a woman turning 40 goes. As much as we'd like to believe otherwise, things *do* start to fall apart.

The big 4-0 is a wonderful time in a woman's life. The children don't need you always and you finally have that much needed time for yourself. You can keep your date with the girlfriends without worrying about your child's homework or tell your husband to fend for himself for a night and not worry about how he'll react. But this age also brings with it BIG problems. This is the time when the body—one that has served you so well all these years—goes into transition. In a certain sense, it is the beginning of the second half of your life. If you look at it in medical terms, you're stepping from a low-risk zone into a high-risk one.

It's an age that can be pretty hard to handle because you're not older—at least in your mind you aren't. Some of you don't look it either. The first thing I ask patients when they come to my clinic is their age because that's a big part of diagnosing. The moment they step in, I play a little game in my head where I try and guess their age. I should've stopped playing a long time ago because I almost never get it right. My mind says '35' but she says '45'.

The one reason why I've wanted to write this book is because there aren't many books dedicated to women of this age. There are hundreds of books in the market on pregnancy, diet, and how to look good, but not many that help a woman make a successful and stress-free transition to the second half of her life. Also, everyone caters to the younger woman. Magazines and advertising budgets keep younger women in mind while developing their products. Very little focus is given to women in their 40s.

For the most part, the 40s have been a neglected phase. Though I must admit that a lot has been written about full-blown menopause, I still feel that women who aren't suffering from menopause and don't have babies have a different set of issues that need to be addressed. For example, very few people know what sort of contraception a woman in her 40s should use. Topics like this are never discussed because being pregnant at 40 is considered a reckless thing to do. The most common reaction in that scenario would be, 'Doesn't she know enough at this age to avoid an unplanned pregnancy?'

While you may not feel or look older, the body's wear-and-tear goes on silently for years. And no one visits a gynaecologist till there's a problem. When I tell older women who I meet socially that I am a gynaecologist, they say they don't need me anymore because they're done planning their family. But you need your gynaecologist at every stage, especially after you cross 40, because that's when you're more prone to health issues like uterine prolapse, problems of abnormal menstrual bleeding, and cancers.

WHY IS 40 A LANDMARK AGE?

Then why am I writing about just the 40s? That's because after puberty, this is the time you see the maximum changes in your body. Sooner or later, you'll suffer from several issues that'll have you question your mental strength, your ability to withstand the ravages of time and, at times, your sanity. You are likely to face problems you've never encountered before in your life. You'll realize that your body is not the way it used to be. You're more vulnerable to diseases and your ability to recover from them isn't the same either.

But it's important to remember that not everyone faces the same problems. A lot depends on how you've lived your life so far. I'm in my 40s. For me, turning 40 has been a positive experience. My fifth decade started off with a huge party my husband threw for me. The only problem I faced was a nagging backache that got worse in my 40s. Since the pain refused to go away, I decided to have a spinal surgery done. There were some post-operative problems. I developed deep vein thrombosis, a life-threatening complication especially because I could not take blood thinning agents to treat it as it could lead to bleeding in the spine. This usually happens to obese, old ladies, which I was not. I was slim and 40 but that is how life is! What can happen will happen, so I decided I will not let it affect me. Some bed rest, physiotherapy, medication and I was back on my feet and raring to go.

There was also the usual weight issue. I've always been a very slim person, but after turning 40, I've had to work towards maintaining my weight. I've become more particular about my workouts and what I eat. Weight gain is a big concern for women over 40 because the rate of metabolism slows down and your body tends to retain a lot more of the fat that it did when you were younger. But more on that later.

As I said before, 40s are when you're more settled and don't have to keep a constant tab on your partner and children. The same applies for me as well. My husband and I recently moved into our own home with the kids after living with my in-laws for years. I definitely feel much more settled now than when I was just starting out as a doctor. The main reason why I think I'm handling this phase of my life so well is acceptance—accepting that life has changed—and being okay with the changes. The fact that I will never be a 20-year-old—and thank God for it—is something I remind myself every day so I can avoid the trap of self-loathing.

If you don't make these mental adjustments, you're very likely to be depressed all the time and you'll continue to try, and fail to look like you're in your mid-20s. Trust me when I tell you that as long as you feel fit and healthy, you're fine. A little bit of imperfection is what makes us stand out. Fortunately, not all of us are Bollywood stars and our body is not our ticket to success. So if your waist is 2 inches more than when you were in your 20s, it shouldn't bother you.

Hollywood actor Halle Berry very wisely said, 'A magical thing happened when I turned 40—a light sort of went off, and I felt more self-assured and confident, like I finally had the right to be authentic about who I am, to say what I want to say. I guess that comes with getting older.' There's no reason why this can't apply to you as well.

How is 40 different from 30 and 50?

Being 28 and being 32 is more or less the same thing. You pretty much live the same life at that time. But there's a lot of difference in being 38 and being 42. As I said before, in your 40s, your body starts to shift gears in a new direction. While that's an internal thing, people around you also start treating you differently. You are suddenly being called 'aunty' by everyone. And, more importantly, the attitude of your doctor changes. Even in the medical field, we categorize 40 as the turning point. You would typically start your cancer screening at 40. This is not to say that you don't get cancer at a younger age. But 40 is a reasonable age for a woman to get her mammogram because that is the age when the chances of breast cancer increase. It's also a good time to start your annual health check-up.

Fifty, meanwhile, is a different ball game altogether. Menopause has finally set in and all the symptoms you experienced as a 40-year-old will now show their true colours. Of course, this does not apply to all women. But for most of us, it holds true.

If someone tells me the reason why they became a doctor when they started out was to help people every day, I'll point out a show-off. But as I've grown older, I've realized that we really have the power to do that. Not just as a surgeon, but also by getting across more information about the complex female body so women can make better decisions for themselves.

Yes, it's true that certain things may never happen at 40. It is unlikely that your secret dream of playing a Bollywood diva will materialize, just as the likelihood of dancing the night away without paying for it the next day fades. While you cannot turn back time, turning 40 suggests something exciting. The word 'turning' means you can turn into anything you want to be. It also means you can turn on your best self, turn the page, and move on.

If you're like most women, you've probably spent your life focussing on the people who need you—your husband, your children, and your parents. But now, it's time to bring the focus back on yourself.

How to Use this Book

FOR SOME REASON, OUR CULTURE has conditioned us to believe that turning 40 is the beginning of the end. For some women, their 40th birthday is a dreaded and unwanted day. Irrespective of what I've said above, your 40th birthday should be a time to celebrate all the good things you've done in your life and make plans to do even bigger and better things.

And all of that begins with a healthier you. This book aims to help you take that step of awareness. When you know better, you do better. And by the time you're done reading this book, you'll have all the information you need to take a confident, healthy, assured step into the next phase of your life. Despite the information at our disposal, our body remains a mystery for most of us. We know very little about how changing hormone levels affect our brain, our bones, our heart, our vulnerability to diseases—and what we should be doing about it.

Part 1, Thinking 40, talks about the physical, emotional, and social changes that'll happen as you cross this age and how you can combat them while keeping your sanity. Part 2, Feeling 40, talks of the major gynaecological conditions that concern women after 40 like bleeding, fibroids, and uterine prolapse. And finally, Part 3, Fit at 40, will give you information about the diseases to look out for and the check-ups that should be on the top of your to-do list. The chapter on exercise, written by Leena Mongre, shows you why it is important to exercise as we cross 40, and also gives you tips to a fab body. Your diet is always important, but it is even more important during menopause. The chapter on diet by Dr Sarita Davare, a weight loss and fitness expert, highlights how, with a minor tweak in your diet, your fitness can be at its optimum best. The final chapter on anti-ageing by dermatologist Purnima Mhatre shows you the causes for skin ageing and the ways to reverse back the clock.

Part 1

Thinking 40

'When I turned 40, I was like, huh.
I accept myself more now.
It was much more comforting.'

—Jennifer Lopez

It is no secret that as we age, our bodies undergo various changes. The changes in middle age tend to be detrimental to our health. Whenever we hit an age that marks a decade (20, 30, 40), we cross an important threshold. Remember when you thought that your life, as you knew it, had ended after you'd reached 30? Well, 40 is the *real* deal. And the reason for that are hormones, more specifically, the hormone oestrogen. Everything that happens in your body after you turn 40 can be safely blamed on hormones. They affect your weight, your mood, and your desire for sex, among many other things. For many women turning 40 can be smooth sailing, but for others it can be a shipwreck at every turn. For some it gets so overwhelming that they feel like they have lost control of their life. The lead-up to the midlife transition can be a scary time. Your changing hormones can set off any number of symptoms that vary from woman to woman. This unpredictability can be shocking and unsettling, especially if you think you're too young for these changes.

So what are these changes that take place when a woman turns 40, and what effect can they have on her health? The book will tackle all these changes you can expect to take place in your body. Some of these changes can be modified, others controlled. But none can be avoided altogether. The important thing is to realize which is which and pick your battles.

1

Physical Changes

Starting in our late 40s and continuing into our 50s, women go into perimenopause, in which estrogen levels begin to decline. Perimenopause means 'around menopause' and refers to the time period during which a woman's body makes its natural transition toward permanent infertility or menopause. While, by definition, menopause is when you don't have your period for one year, women can be perimenopausal for several years. It can begin as early as the mid-30s or as late as the 50s for some women. Most often it starts during the mid to late 40s. A 2010 study by the Indian Menopause Society shows that the menopausal age among urban women across the country is between 47 and 52 years.

Perimenopause also signals the decline of oestrogen levels in your body. This primary female sex hormone is responsible for a lot of positive things. It performs over 400 functions in the body, ranging from taking care of your skin, maintaining the density of your bones, reducing anxiety and depression, regulating your menstrual cycle, and giving strength to all the tissues. It is only after the oestrogen levels decline, as you turn 40, that everything starts to weaken. Studies over the years that have shown that oestrogen also protects women from heart attacks, which is why they don't suffer from it as often as men do. But that's only before menopause. After menopause, a woman is as much at risk of a heart attack as a man.

During perimenopause, oestrogen levels fluctuate, triggering switches in your menstrual cycle—they may be lighter, shorter, heavier, or longer. Irregular ovulation makes it much more difficult to get pregnant. While two-thirds of women over 40 experience fertility problems, those who do become pregnant also face a higher risk of complications like diabetes during pregnancy, miscarriage, hypertension, etc.

Weight gain

A woman in her early 40s came to my clinic one day and exclaimed, 'I have been slim all my life and I am doing exactly what I used to do, but I am still putting on weight, particularly around the middle.' This is a common complaint among woman in the age group of 40–50. Weight gain at this time is one of the effects of dropping levels of oestrogen. It's a big concern because the rate of metabolism slows down as you age. Metabolism is the process by which your body converts what you eat and drink into energy. When you're younger, this process takes place at a much rapid pace. But as you grow older, the amount of muscle tends to decrease and fat accounts for most of your weight, slowing down the calorie burning process. Simply put, it's easier to pile on the kilos after 40 than when you were younger because of the decrease in metabolism. As your ovaries produce less oestrogen, the body attempts to find the hormones in places other than the ovaries. Fat cells can produce oestrogen, so your body works harder to convert calories into fat to increase oestrogen levels. Unfortunately, fat cells don't burn calories the way muscle cells do, which causes weight gain. The only way out seems to exercise more than you used to and eat half of what you did earlier to maintain your weight. But this, as we all know, is very, very difficult.

In the 40s, most doctors recommend that you do moderate aerobic activity like brisk walking, for at least 150 minutes a week, or vigorous aerobic activity like jogging, for at least 75 minutes a week. And this is just to maintain weight. Strength training exercises are recommended at least twice a week. If you want to lose weight or meet specific fitness goals, you might need to exercise more. Another simple-to-advise-but-difficult-to-implement rule is to eat less. To maintain your current weight —forget losing the excess kilos—you will need about 200 lesser calories a day during your perimenopausal years. To reduce calories without affecting your nutrition, you have to watch what you're eating and drinking. Eat more fruits, vegetables, and whole grains. Read the chapter on Diet on page 182 to know more.

'Belly fat expands as we age,' says Dr Mehmet Oz, Oprah Winfrey's go-to doctor for everything. 'This is tied to an increased production of cortisol, the stress hormone. Combined with other hormonal factors such as low androgens, fat cells become inflamed and tissues expand to create fat where you want it least—around your middle. Called omentum, this blubbery tissue pumps out chemicals that keep you fat, creating a vicious cycle and potential health issues you can't hide from, even with an oversized kaftan.'[1]

Try as you may, there's no escaping that you are going to weigh more as you grow older. Take a look at your pictures from five years ago. Chances are you'll look a bit rounder now. You are always going to weigh more at 30 than you did at 20. But it's at 40 that the weight really hits you. After the age of 40, the rules change, and you cannot eat the way you did when you were 30. That's because a 40-year-old woman has a very different body than she had 10 years earlier. It's a typical Indian trait to put on weight in the middle. That's also why we're more susceptible to diabetes and heart diseases. One of the reasons why we're more vulnerable to diseases is our culture. We, as a race, aren't very physical. When was the last time you consciously made an effort to run? I'm guessing it was on your annual sports day at school, isn't it? From a young age, we've been trained to spend our free time studying. So we've never gotten into the habit of running.

Weight gain in the 40s also means flabby arms and a wrinkled neck. Three in four women hate the fat that accumulates in their upper arms, which is also known as 'bingo wings'. A 2010 survey by British magazine *Prima* found that one in four bingo wings sufferers were so embarrassed by their flabby upper arms that they had stopped waving in public![2] The only solution is to hit the gym and lift weights or give up your dream of going sleeveless. A wrinkled neck is also difficult to camouflage. No amount of exercise will revert the havoc of ageing on your neck. A late pregnancy is also another reason for weight gain in your 40s. It pains me to say this, but our mums were right. It's better to marry early and have your kids early so your body doesn't suffer much. I've always told my patients to take their time and have children when they're ready. But now I've realized that it's practical to keep your age in mind before you subject your body to a lot of change.

LOSS OF BLADDER CONTROL

Involuntary discharge of urine is not something we ever thought would affect us—unless we were on our deathbed. It is a subject many of us find too embarrassing to talk about, leading many women to suffer in silence. Women who've had normal deliveries, suddenly realize after 40 that they are unable to control their bladder. Sometimes, this happens when they cough, sneeze, laugh, or exercise. This is known as Stress Urinary Incontinence (SUI). It is more common in women who've had normal deliveries than those who had a planned caesarean section because of the stretching and sometimes tearing of the vagina and pelvis supports. You don't face this problem when your hormones are working fine. But with age, things aren't the same anymore. Sometimes because of the stretching and loosening of the pelvic floor due to normal deliveries, repetitive strenuous work, or inherited tissue weakness, there is weakening of the support of the urinary outlet tube (urethra). A simple gynaecological examination on a full bladder by your doctor can clinch the diagnosis. There are specific tests, such as urodynamic testing—a study that assesses how the bladder and urethra are performing their job of storing and releasing urine—which can differentiate SUI from irritable bladder or failure of the valve mechanism of the urethra. So whenever there is increased pressure due to coughing or sneezing, the urine leaks out. Lowered oestrogen level means that muscle pressure around your urethra is weaker and leaks are more likely to occur. This may result in a feeling of wetness and continuous urine smell from your undergarments.

Hot flashes

There is a lot of difference in how women react to ageing. Some women suffer menopause, others just let it pass by without a worry. Everyone has different symptoms and their ability to handle these symptoms is different as well. I've observed that at times women who don't pay much heed to the changes happening in their body deal with the situation much better. Other women who know a lot more about menopausal changes have much more acute reactions. Such women are generally very focused on hot flashes.

Hot flashes are sudden feelings of warmth that are most intense over the face, neck, and chest. Your skin may redden, just as if you were blushing. They can also cause profuse sweating and may leave you feeling chilled. The skin's temperature rises, then falls, and is accompanied by heart palpitations, nausea, and anxiety. Hot flashes are one of the earliest symptoms of menopause, although they can also be caused by other hormonal conditions. Depending on the person, hot flashes can occur a few times a week or several times a day. Research has shown that three out of four women experience hot flashes.

Most hot flashes happen during the night. It's not uncommon for women to feel extremely hot even though they're sleeping in an air-conditioned environment. Sometimes, though, they happen during the day. That's when they get embarrassing. Unfortunately, sometimes hot flashes go on for years on end. They can last for about six months to a year, but other times they do go on for much, much longer. This happens because there is a transition in the hormones. And for women who suffer from hot flashes the longest, the transition is not very smooth.

Indian women, traditionally and culturally, aren't open to sharing what they're going through. One of the main reasons for that is lack of information. When you don't know enough about a problem, you tend to think you're the only one suffering from it. And why add to your embarrassment by talking about it with someone else? That's why I loved that episode from the last season of the cult show, *Sex and the City*. One of the leads, Samantha Jones, who's also in her 40s, has breast cancer and is perimenopausal. She gives a speech for a cancer benefit dinner, and while on stage, she starts suffering from hot flashes. She remains tight-lipped about it because she doesn't want anyone to know. But it gets too much for her to take after a while and she removes her wig on stage, admitting that she is suffering from hot flashes. The audience appreciates her honesty and gives her a standing ovation. How I wish I met more women like Samantha in India. Women who aren't ashamed of their new body and willingly embrace their changes.

I used to work with a doctor in one of the larger hospitals of Mumbai. A couple of years ago, I came out of surgery one day and found her sitting outside her OT, literally dripping in sweat. I asked her if she was okay and she embarrassingly confessed that she had been suffering from terrible hot flashes. I've known so many women who have bad bouts of hot flashes, but none was as bad as hers. At one point, she was squeezing sweat from her handkerchief. She was suffering so much, while she was at work! She had taken a small break to deal with her hot flashes and wanted to go back to work as soon as she felt a little better. I wrote her some medication to give her temporary relief. We got to talking after that and she told me that perimenopause had been very difficult for her. Unfortunately, at the same time, she was going through a crisis because a patient of hers had suffered from major medical complications and she was very stressed about it.

A few days after the episode, came the grave news that the doctor had committed suicide. To say that I was shocked would not do justice to the gravity of my feelings. She wasn't a gynaecologist, but I had worked with her on and off on several cases. The problem with her patient, coupled with terrible menopausal symptoms, clearly must've driven her to suicide. And as I gathered later, she had been depressed for a long time. Her only daughter had just gotten married and she was feeling lonely by herself. So she was probably in a fragile situation and difficult and uncomfortable menopausal symptoms must have just tipped her over the edge.

This incident is, of course, an extreme form of perimenopause. But it shows us that we can't take the changes and problems that women of a certain age go through lightly. What I've noticed is that women resign themselves to the changes as they grow older. It's not uncommon for me to hear sentences like, 'I am going through menopause, so I will have to suffer through hot flashes and mood swings.' A lot of women have that carefree attitude. But it does not have to be that way. After what happened with my former colleague, I know now that no woman should take problems like depression and illnesses lightly. It's extremely important to give them the attention that's due. Recognition of the problem is the most important thing. This was not the first time my doctor colleague was breaking out into hot flashes. If only someone had bothered enough to advise her to see a gynaecologist, things could have been different.

ASIAN WOMEN SUFFER LESS

It has been observed that women in some cultures—mostly Asian—rarely experience discomfort from hot flashes. Several studies suggest that there may be cultural and biological differences in whether women experience hot flashes. An American study found that few Indian women report any problems with menopause other than changes in cyclicity, and reporting of hot flashes by Japanese women is lower than that by women in Western cultures. Diet is one of the main reasons for that.[4] Research indicates that soy, a significant ingredient in the Japanese diet, may be useful in preventing hot flashes in women.

In addition to soy products, you can help fight hot flashes by eating more calcium- and magnesium-rich foods and foods rich in Vitamin E like green leafy vegetables, nuts, and almonds, as well as plenty of mineral- and fibre-rich foods like whole grains.

Osteoporosis

As a woman gradually nears actual menopause, bone degeneration becomes a major issue. Osteopenia, which is weakness of the bone, or osteoporosis, which is the absolute erosion of the bone density, sets in. This may not happen with everyone. If you are entering menopause with good bone strength, it will be enough to pull you through. But if you're entering it with fairly weak bones, which unfortunately happens to almost all women these days, then there is a rapid decline in bone strength. This decline in oestrogen causes an accelerated rate of bone loss. This rapid loss of bone continues for about 10 years after menopause. This causes postmenopausal women to have a much greater chance of having a fracture. Osteoporosis is so severe that the normal stress on bones from sitting, standing, coughing, or even hugging can result in painful fractures and immobility. The scary part is that there are no symptoms of this bone disease until you fracture a bone. The most common sites of fracture after osteoporosis sets in are the radius (wrist), the spine, and the hip. As a younger woman, a fracture is just that—a fracture, but in a menopausal woman a fracture can be life-threatening. The spine, in the meantime, undergoes very subtle fractures, whereby it compresses. Women with severe osteoporosis of the spine, walk with a very pronounced stoop. Most spinal compression fractures are never diagnosed because many patients think that back pain is merely a sign of ageing and arthritis.

There's also the usual joint and knee pain, and the heels begin to hurt. It may seem insignificant, but not being able to wear heels can be upsetting for a woman who's always been out and about. I've seen a lot of women in their 40s opting for more comfortable footwear. At a party recently, I met my friend who had come wearing flats. Her choice of footwear was a surprise for me because in so many years of knowing her, I had never seen her in anything but heels. That night at the party, she told me, 'Forget heels; it's not about style anymore. It's all about comfort.'

DID YOU KNOW?

At least one in three women in India suffer from an osteoporotic fracture during their lifetime. Studies show that a 50-year-old woman has a similar lifetime risk of dying from hip fracture as from breast cancer.[5] As per a data furnished in International Osteoporosis Foundation, experts peg the number of osteoporosis patients in India at approximately 2.6 crore in 2003. That number is projected to increase to 3.6 crore by 2013. More than half of these are women in their 40s and above.[6]

AGEING OF SKIN

During your 40s, the body is undergoing profound changes, and the skin is no different. It is a time where dryness can exist simultaneously with acne. I have many patients in their 40s who say, 'I now have wrinkles. So why am I still getting acne?' Unfortunately, because of fluctuating hormone levels, acne around the mouth and jawline is quite common in the 40s. Then comes the most common problem—wrinkles. If you haven't seen one already, you are likely to see your first wrinkle in your 40s. Genetics, sun exposure, and your skin-care routine contribute to how the skin ages. The loss of hormones causes a decline in the synthesis of collagen and elastin, reduces the production of sebum (skin oil), and leads to skin thinning and dryness. You can see the signs of ageing even on a woman who has maintained herself well. You cannot run away from the fact that your skin is going to show some amount of wrinkling—whether it's the forehead or the crow's feet around the eyes or the nasal folds. The tightness of the skin, which comes naturally when you're younger, withers away slowly after you cross the 40 mark.

Most wrinkles can be treated with Botox injections. That's, of course, after you've tried other, simple solutions. Botox is snake venom in a very diluted form. Frowning, and hence frown lines, is caused by the spasming and relaxing of certain muscles. Botox is injected into contracting muscles that result in a frown. When injected, it paralyses the muscle where you use it. So the skin will remain relaxed and won't cause wrinkles. Botox works well for lines on the forehead, crow's feet, and corner of the lips. Of course, because it's a drug, its effect will wear away eventually and you'll have to redo the procedure in about 6–7 months. If done the right way, Botox will not give you that typical flat look.

You have to remember that the type of skin you have is genetic. You can't turn horrible skin into fantastic. But if it's a hormone-related problem, you can turn it around. Acne, for example, can be treated with hormones. Hormones that were erratic when you were an adolescent, hence causing acne, are likely to behave equally erratic when you are in your 40s. That's why a lot of women break out into adult acne. It's usually more common on the chin. Adult acne tends to respond well to antibiotics. Multiple, short courses of antibiotics are seen to work well for adult acne.

A lot of women also have coarse hair on their chin in their 40s. This can be blamed on the male hormones working actively. The problem could be because of a disease—an ovarian tumour could be secreting testosterone. Or it may be hormonal—your ovaries secrete more male hormones than they usually do. Your adrenaline gland also could be on an overdrive and secrete more male hormone. Hormonal problems like these can be treated with a combination of drugs. Of course, the facial hair needs to be treated cosmetically. But subsequent hair growth will be much lighter and finer after treatment. In your 40s, there is also a lot of loss of fat under the cheeks. That results in a sunken face because you cheeks don't look as pumped as when you were younger.

Pigmentation is another aspect of ageing. Patchy pigmentation across the nose and cheeks is quite common.

Visible ageing as against the changes happening inside your body is much more difficult to handle, probably because evidence that you're not young any more, looks back at you in the mirror every day. How you cope with ageing depends on your patience, confidence, and how you're coping with the other changes your body is going through.

CHANGES IN HAIR

With age, your hair undergoes major changes too. Greying, of course, starts early these days, may be even in the 20s and 30s. But as with most things related to ageing, it hits you most in the 40s. Natural changes that occur over time—like the loss of cellular reproduction, hormone changes, and diet—can all impact the health of your hair. The effect of natural oils that lubricate the scalp, hair, and skin reduces because of age. But it won't be right to attribute greying of hair to menopause. Everyone is greying prematurely these days and a whole lot of factors are responsible for it. Our parents and grandparents greyed much later in life. But today even girls in their 20s have significant grey hair. There isn't any direct connection between change in hormones and grey hair. It is more an ageing process rather than hormonal. Greying has a lot more to do with genetics– if your parents greyed at 40, you are definitely going to go grey earlier. Environment, chemicals, and stress—all wreak havoc on your hair.

Hair thinning is psychologically traumatic for a woman.

To see thinning hair where there used to be a full head of hair is not an easy change to accept. Some people are quick to brush off these concerns as superficial and accuse you of being conceited about your looks. But it's very easy to judge someone, especially when you aren't undergoing these changes.

Hormones play a huge role in hair fall and thinning. Oestrogen, as it is for most things, is very good for the hair. It's responsible for the thickness of the hair and ensures less hair fall. During pregnancy, there are a lot of hormones in the body and you see that the hair is really thick and glossy. And then when the hormone levels fall following delivery, women suffer from hair loss. And you realize this only once you hit 40 because before that the body is well-equipped to heal itself. Similarly, during perimenopause, one of the most common complaints is hair thinning and drying which is related to a severe decline in the levels of oestrogen over a period of time. Decline of oestrogen can also cause hair to become dryer, coarser, and a lot less shiny. If you have thyroid issues, the situation worsens. Hypothyrodism is known to cause significant hair fall. Women who are fond of colouring their hair on a regular basis have to face problems of hair damage due to the presence of chemicals.

The most common and best answer to hair fall is a medication called Minoxidil. It is available in the form of solution, gel, and foam, and has to be applied directly on the scalp. It has been documented that Minoxidil is the proven drug to reduce hair fall. It controls the hair cycle and recruits more cells in the growth phase of the hair. It has very few side-effects, but you have to use it long-term for the results to really show.

There are also multivitamin solutions that you apply on your scalp. The scalp has very good blood supply, so any medication you apply there gets absorbed into the body very quickly. An oral supplement of a B-vitamin called biotin is also known to reduce hair fall. Vitamin E is also helpful. One way to camouflage thinning hair is to put fibre dust into your hair so it can camouflage the patches on your scalp. This is available abroad and many hair clinics in India are also now marketing this dark coarse powder, which though expensive, gives a good cosmetic look If all else fails, there's always hair transplant you can fall back on. The most common way to do that is to take hair from the nape of your hair, split each hair into 3-4 hair and implant it. The fact that there are many hair transplant clinics mushrooming all over India is proof that people are very sensitive to hair loss.

LOSS OF VISION

If you're over 40, you've probably noticed your vision has changed. The age-related loss of near focusing ability usually develops at this time. Called presbyopia, you're likely to experience blurred near vision when reading or working on the computer. Even if you're one of those who's always had good eyesight, you still can't escape presbyopia. People who are nearsighted will find that their near vision blurs when they wear their glasses. A common symptom of presbyopia is that when you perform work that's near your eyes, you may develop headaches or your eyes may feel strained or tired. This is a problem both men and women face. When you develop presbyopia, you need to hold all reading material like books, newspapers, and menus at arm's length in order to focus properly.

Menopausal women have another set of eye-related problems caused by ageing. There are some theories that indicate that a decline in the hormone androgen could be the reason for dry eyes. Studies show that about 7.8 percent women and about 4.7 percent men in their 40s and above, suffer from dry eyes.

A more severe problem is the complete loss of vision. While I was hard-pressed to find such studies conducted in India, a study by Prevent Blindness America found that more women than men have age-related macular degeneration, cataracts, glaucoma, and diabetic retinopathy. These are the four leading eye diseases in the world.[7] That's why most doctors recommend that every woman, especially those who are 40 and older, should get a dilated eye exam done. Through early detection, vision loss can be lessened.

Answer the questions below:

- Do you have trouble adjusting to dark rooms?
- Do you face difficulty focusing on objects?
- Do lines and edges appear distorted or wavy?
- Do you squint due to sensitivity to light or glare?

- Are you seeing spots?
- Do you see a change in the colour of your iris?
- Is there recurrent pain in or around your eyes?
- Do you have double vision?
- Do you have dry eyes with itching or burning? Or watery eyes?

If your answer is 'yes' to any of these problems, please visit you eye doctor immediately.

SLOW METABOLISM

You've been exercising regularly, you watch what you eat, but your weight still remains the same. Do you know what is to blame? A decline in your metabolism rate. Women over 40 tend to gradually lose healthy muscle mass and bone density and have decreased metabolism. This is the reason why you don't lose as much weight as you did when you were in your 20s and 30s.

So what is metabolism? It is the rate at which your body burns calories. Calories are burnt even when you're sleeping and eating, because you need energy to keep you going. But it differs for every woman. That explains why the diet and exercise regimen your partner or best friend follows may not work for you. Factors such as muscle mass, genetics, overall weight, age and fat content determine how fast or slow your metabolism is.

What then influences your metabolism?

There are some factors that you can control and change, and some factors that you can't.

Age: After 40, metabolism naturally slows down. Your metabolic rate decreases by 5 percent with each decade.

Gender: Men generally burn calories more quickly than women because they have more muscle tissue.

Heredity: You can inherit your metabolic rate.

Thyroid disorder: Hypothyroidism and hyperthyroidism can slow down or speed up metabolism. According to the American thyroid association women are 5–8 times more likely than men to have a thyroid disorder. One in eight women will develop a thyroid disorder in her lifetime, so a test for thyroid should always be done if you are facing weight issues.

This accounts, at least partially, for the weight gain that comes with ageing. Speeding up your metabolism after 40 takes some work, but it can be done.

How do you rev it up?

Eat sensible, eat healthy, eat often: Spacing out your meals too much can lead to cravings and a drop in blood sugar level. To keep your glucose steady and your metabolism working at its maximum capacity, eat small meals every

3–4 hours, rather than just a few big ones. Eat small meals often rather than big meals far apart. Try to eat 4–6 small meals and snacks daily. Most people think that the thinner a person, the better their metabolic rate is, and that this gives her a licence to go on a junk food binge. Junk food, oily, and spicy food can slow down metabolism because these foods are tougher to digest and they add more to the fat content than to energy levels. That being said, you can still add spicy foods like jalapeno peppers to your diet. These peppers contain capsaicin, a chemical that boosts metabolism and increases calorie burning for up to 3 hours after you've finished your meal.

Exercise: It hikes your metabolism level simply because your body needs to burn more calories to sustain itself during and after a workout. Most people try to lose weight by doing a lot of cardiovascular exercises like running. However, adding some weight-training increases your metabolism because muscles require a lot of calories to sustain themselves. Women should exercise for at least 30 minutes daily from their late 20s onwards because metabolism slows down considerably after that. The more muscle tissue you have, the more calories you will burn even while you're resting or sleeping. An increased metabolism also helps in faster digestion; so if you work out, even an occasional heavy meal does not make you feel bloated like it normally would. Exercise can also help reduce the chance of other health problems that are common after 40, such as heart disease. Hiking and running are especially helpful. Strength training helps build muscle, which in turn speeds up metabolism. Women tend to do more cardio exercises because they think only these help in weight loss. But lifting weights and building muscle mass also helps burn calories and causes weight loss. If you're looking to rev up your metabolism, ask for specific strength training workouts, apart from putting in more time on the treadmill and cross-trainer.

Sleep: Women who sleep less than 7 hours a night cause their systems to slow down the next day—their reflexes becomes sluggish and food is digested slowly. Women over 40 usually find that they have more trouble falling and staying asleep because of perimenopause. Meditation or yoga can help the body relax and get more consistent sleep.

Eat the right foods: Some foods are difficult to digest and so consume more calories in the digestive process. Eating these foods will help your body to burn more calories naturally. These include high protein foods like cod and trout, and fruits and vegetables like apples, berries, celery, and grapes. You can also have oatmeal and whole grains.

Change in libido

Oestrogen plays an important role in female sexuality though its exact role is not known. It is known to help cause vaginal lubrication, and maintain the health of vaginal tissues. As the production of oestrogen reduces during menopause, a woman will begin to feel a loss of sexual desire. Progesterone hormones are also integral to maintaining sexual health. When the levels of progesterone become too low during menopause, the resulting irregular periods, fatigue, and other menopause symptoms can cause loss of libido. Perimenopause is associated with a decline of estrogen, as well as androgens. And this is believed to account for the lowered levels of sexual desire and motivation in older women, although the direct relationship is not well understood.

Nowadays, women are more open to talking about sex and the problems that come with it. Most women are unfortunately not in sync with men as far as sexual desire is concerned. In her book *The Sex Starved Marriage*, American psychologist Michele Weiner Davis says that one in every three married couples struggle with problems associated with mismatched libidos—that men want sex more than their wives.[8] This problem is more pronounced in the 40s. And that results in a number of conflicts between the couple. A large majority of my patients who are in their 40s have told me that they have no desire for sex anymore. Though most men have as high a libido as they did in their younger days, it's not the case with older women.

I had a patient who'd been suffering from vaginal infections for a long time. I was unable to understand why she was getting repeated infections, so I decided to conduct a couple of extra tests for her. We eventually found out that she had an HPV infection, which is a sexually transmitted disease. She was very upset because she believed that she was in a monogamous relationship. She then confessed that she has no desire to have sex and was forcing herself to have sex because her husband wanted it. The sad part is that she spoke about having no desire for sex only after we diagnosed her infection. This shows that some women aren't very forthcoming about their non-existent desire for sex because they are embarrassed by it.

Unfortunately, there's very little we can do to increase sexual desire, other than actually giving women testosterone. There used to be a time when doctors did give women testosterone in the form of a patch or by injecting it. But it's not freely available now because it has side-effects like hair growth on the face and voice changes. You can, of course, opt for counselling, but that may or may not work. Recently, a clitoral gel has been introduced in the market. It doesn't increase sexual desire as such, but makes the nerve endings at the clitoris more sensitive as well as helps in increasing the blood supply to the region. I'm glad that finally pharma companies are bringing out such products keeping the woman's satisfaction in mind.

The synthetic compound sildenaphil, better known as Viagra, taken to enhance male potency can also be taken by women. It also increases the supply of blood to the vagina and clitoris. So women can use Viagra with the same precautions that men do. Women with a history of heart disease, blood pressure, or headaches must consult a physician before taking Viagra. Dropping oestrogen levels also mean less vaginal lubrication, which can make sexual intercourse difficult and painful. After menopause, the vagina actually shrinks. The vaginal lining becomes very thin and sometimes even tears. In this case, you can also use the plain old lubricating gel because vaginal dryness is a major issue.

Vaginal oestrogen creams are also available, which, when used for a few weeks, improve lubrication.

GRAB AN EROTICA!

There's a reason why the erotic novel *50 Shades Of Grey* is such a hit with older women. Called 'mummy porn' in honour of women over 40 who turned out to be the trilogy's biggest fans, the book has sold over 1 crore copies worldwide. So what is it about the book that has women over 40 so excited? A lot of women have much lowered sex drives as we age and the fact that our focus has shifted to other responsibilities, it takes longer to warm up to sex. We need to be led into it, whether it's through being romanced, or reading some good ol' erotica.

2

Cognitive Changes

HAVE YOU HEARD THE OLD saying, 'Change is the only constant?' There's no guarantee that we'll behave today the way we did yesterday. What seems like boring behaviour in the 20s can suddenly be perceived as mature and responsible when you are in your 30s. So when we change the way we think without any external pressures, can you imagine what happens when your body makes the mind dance to its tunes? That is what the 40s are all about. When you don't have much control over how you react and the frustrations it brings, you know that you have reached a place in your life where turning back the clock becomes virtually impossible. Acceptance is half the battle won and the rest is all about holding your nerve.

Fatigue

This is a very common symptom in menopause. Forty-plus women often complain of lack of energy, and feeling tired and weak. Our hormones are responsible for controlling energy at the cellular level in our body and so an oestrogen and progesterone deficiency after 40 will definitely cause a loss of energy. Also, changes in thyroid and adrenal hormones have a role to play in fatigue. As menopause may affect sleep, the woman is more exhausted due to lack of a good night's sleep. This is exacerbated by frequent hot flashes at night which wakes them up or even disturbs sleep due to snoring or restless leg syndrome (RLS)—a neurological disorder that causes unpleasant sensations in the leg, leading to an uncontrollable urge to move them. This, of course, ruins her day, as the woman is fatigued, depressed, or anxious and cannot concentrate during the day due to lack of a restful sleep. This can be a vicious cycle.

The only way out is to improve your diet with additional fruits, vegetables, and vitamins, regular exercise, and alternative medicines (such as natural oestrogens in soya extracts). Foods rich in iron, which enriches your blood—like spinach, apricots, and raisins—are great to fight fatigue. Reducing caffeine and alcohol intake, consuming less liquid from evening onwards, avoiding sleeping in the day, and practising yoga are guaranteed to help you. All these tips definitely help get better sleep at night. For women suffering from severe night sweats, low dose hormone replacement therapy may help.

> **DID YOU KNOW?**
>
> 16 percent of postmenopausal women have difficulty falling asleep and 40 percent have disturbed sleep at night.

Memory loss

Remember the time you went looking for your reading glasses only to have your son or daughter tell you they are perched on your head! Such incidents are funny in retrospect. But memory loss is no joke and can cause immense frustration. I can say that from personal experience. There have been so many times when I am about to say something and just can't remember what it was the next minute. Misplacing things has become another common occurrence. With age, many women have trouble remembering names, recent events, phone numbers, and even where their cupboard keys are kept! This happens because of a reduction in oestrogen levels. Lack of sleep and medication may also contribute to memory lapses. A study by the University of Rochester, UK, found that fluctuating levels of female hormones are the likely cause of the problem, which affects women most badly during the first year of the menopause. The study says, 'Parts of the brain most dependent on oestrogen, which diminishes during menopause, are important for verbal memory and processing speed. While absolute hormone levels could not be linked with cognitive function, it is possible that the fluctuations that occur during this time could play a role in the memory problems that many women experience.'[1]

Though there is no specific treatment for memory loss, lifestyle changes with exercise, adequate rest and sleep, avoidance of alcohol and drugs, good nutrition with addition of antioxidants, and intake of vitamins B, C, D, and E are helpful.

The most important thing to remember is that these memory lapses are normal at this stage. I've had patients who, after discovering that it's just a symptom of menopause, are usually very relieved, for they earlier feared it was something worse like Alzheimer's disease.

MIGRAINES

Most women are quick to dismiss migraines as 'just another headache'. But migraine is a particular kind of headache that is concentrated only on one side. They usually start off as headaches near the end of the menstrual cycle when the body's oestrogen levels are low. Not all headaches or migraines are caused by a dip in oestrogen levels, but studies have found that 75 percent of migraines in adults occur in women. Ordinary headaches usually occur near the end of the period, while migraine headaches may also come at the beginning or two days before the start of the period. It is believed that oestrogen controls serotonin in the brain, which controls chemicals that can constrict blood vessels to cause a headache.

During perimenopause, oestrogen levels can be extremely high on some days and then drop to undetectable levels on other days. Women who have never suffered from migraines before may have much worse migraines during this period. Even women who have never had menstrual headaches start to have them during perimenopause. According to the International Headache Society, menstrual migraine can occur any time from two days before a period to the third day of bleeding.[2] These migraines last longer than non-menstrual ones because the underlying trigger—a drop in oestrogen—is there for several days. Interestingly, once a woman reaches menopause and produces much less oestrogen, she stops having hormone-related headaches and migraines.

Contraceptive pills are also known to cause migraines in some patients. This may be due to the estrogen contained in them and possibly due to the water retention which some pills cause. However, the newer pills with ultra low dose hormones and newer progestogens have a much lower incidence of migraines. If a particular pill causes migraine, you can ask your doctor to switch you to a different combination or preparation and a lower dose. Even estrogen-free or progesterone-only pills are also available. Non-hormonal contraceptive choices can also be made. However, the women who suffer from menstrual migraines may actually benefit from contraceptive pills. Birth control pills contain hormones for 21 days followed by 7 pill-free days to allow menstrual bleeding. These women get migraine during the 7 day pill-free interval. For these women it is recommended to take the contraceptive pill continuously for 3 months without a break, and hence without any menstrual period for that time.

Since most women won't associate migraines with their period, I'd advise you to keep a diary, noting each day of your period and marking each day of a migraine attack with a cross. If a cross occurs either on the day of bleeding or the two days either side—and this happens for at least two or three cycles—it is an indication you were suffering from a menstrual migraine. One common way to avoid migraines is to have food that's low on salt. You could also use another type of contraceptive if the birth control pills you've been using regularly are causing your migraines.

3

Psychological Changes

I BELIEVE THAT WOMEN FACE two events that can change their lives forever. The first crisis is adolescence—where the events and changes that take place will define their personalities and the kind of women they'll grow up to be. And the second is turning 40, where again there are drastic changes in the body and every woman will cope with it differently. A study published in the *Journal of Personality and Social Psychology* found that as people reach middle age and beyond, they tend to care more about their work, responsibilities, and those in their lives. Men become less open to meeting new people, but women become more extroverted.[1]

Anxiety, depression, and mood swings are few of the first signs of perimenopausal transitions. Let's take a look at each of them more closely.

ANXIETY

There are many emotional factors particular to perimenopause that can contribute to anxiety. When perimenopause hits, a woman is likely to suffer from anxiety as well as depression. Though anxiety strikes at any time during a woman's life, hormonal changes can produce feelings of anxiety in those going through menopause. Anxiety is a mental state where you worry too much—sometimes persistently—are nervous, and take tension. Women who experience anxiety often can't seem to shake their concerns and worries about everyday events, even though they know that their anxiety is out of proportion and unjustified. You can have difficulty concentrating, trouble relaxing, and feel restless and irritable, which can sometimes lead to severe cases of panic attacks. Changes in oestrogen levels have a direct effect on the neurochemicals serotonin, norepinephrine, dopamine, and melatonin. Since all of these chemicals play an integral role in emotions and mood regulation, oestrogen fluctuations can lead to anxiety during menopause. Other environmental and social factors, like worrying about your child's exam results may worsen this condition. It's not easy to manage this condition and requires lot of family support and understanding, lifestyle changes, and sometimes medication.

For many women who are essentially happy and upbeat, things change quickly and drastically when perimenopause appears. It's a time of emotional distress for them. Because of this, they have a lot more conflicts than usual with the people around them and that creates tension. Some women are even going through a difficult time with their husbands sexually. Because of this, anxiety issues intensify.

Anxiety leads many menopausal women to experience palpitations or rapid heartbeats. We can, as usual, blame low oestrogen levels for this, but the problem may also be aggravated by caffeine, stress, thyroid problems, or heart disease. It is a good idea to visit a physician and have a thorough check-up done if the heartbeat is faster than 100 beats per minute to rule out any cardiac problem. If all your tests are normal then yoga, relaxation techniques, avoiding caffeine, colas, smoking, and alcohol helps reduce episodes of palpitations.

Depression

Women over the age of 40 go through a lot of changes that can result in depression. This doesn't mean that every woman gets depressed after a certain age. After the age of 40, there's a spike in women who are diagnosed with depression as well as many other mental health issues. If your life was already stressful, the physical and emotional changes that typically accompany menopause may be sufficient to send you into a full-blown state of depression.

In menopause, oestrogen can fall to very low levels, causing a sudden dip in mood. Depression is extremely common in this age group due to declining oestrogen levels as well as brain chemicals like serotonin and cortisol that are responsible for how we feel. Physical ill-health and family issues may worsen this situation. A study published in the *Journal of the Indian Academy of Applied Psychology* says: 'Women's reproductive cycle and post-menopause bring fluctuations in mood that include depression. These events may lead to depression by fostering low self-esteem, a sense of helplessness, self-blame, social isolation, and low morale. Depressive illness makes them feel exhausted, worthless, helpless and hopeless, and sometimes develop the feelings to give up. Women often suppress their need of autonomy, neglect their health, and fail to equip with skills, competence, and self-confidence. Lifestyle factors have a greater psychological impact than genetics, which increase longevity, delay illness, and improve the quality of life.'[2]

Women are likely to experience sadness, crying spells, sleeplessness or excessive sleep, fatigue, lack of interest in surroundings, neglect of self, and many other signs of depression which may be as serious as suicide attempts. The treatment consists of lifestyle changes, exercise, yoga, support from family and friends, and many times, anti-depressant drugs.

When you were younger, you could take on a lot more pressure. But as you grow older, your ability to take the stuff life throws at you diminishes. No matter what your age, stress can affect you. Whether it's a student worried about studying, an employee worried about meeting a deadline, or a woman affected by the sudden changes in her body—

everyone worries. But women over 40 are more prone to stress and anxiety. Midlife issues such as menopause, caring for ageing parents, career changes, children leaving home and financial setbacks make ageing women the perfect target for stress related problems. Stress can lead to a number of problems like obesity, heart diseases, digestive problems, disinterest in sex, insomnia, and high blood pressure.

DID YOU KNOW?

Women in perimenopause phase are four times more likely to be depressed than their younger counterparts.

MOOD CHANGES

A change in mood is the most common symptom of perimenopause. Most of us have experienced irritability and mood swings. As a teenager, some of you may have cried at the drop of a hat. As a woman in your 20s and 30s, PMS made you bite your best friend's head off when she asked you how your day went. Or remember that feeling of wanting to punch someone because they just wouldn't shut up when you told them to? Well, that feeling is going to come back to you when you least expect it, in circumstances that wouldn't be classified as volatile. We'd all like to keep these episodes to a minimum, but perimenopause can sometimes make that seem like an impossible challenge.

Depression, anxiety, irrational behaviour, sleeplessness, temper tantrums, irritability, panic attacks, and palpitations are extremely common. Hot flashes, if left unmanaged, can leave you feeling irritable which may eventually lead to mild depression. Women with a history of depression are said to be more prone to experience it during perimenopause and beyond. Perimenopause shares many of these symptoms with that hormone related annoying condition—PMS. The difference is that PMS lasts only for one week, once a month, but perimenopause can last anywhere from 1 to 10 years. It's no wonder that the overriding emotion women in their 40s feel is that of being overwhelmed.

And because you have to train yourself to cope with these feelings, perimonopause also results in a pretty drastic change in a woman's personality. There are days when you don't really know what is happening with you. You'll find yourself annoyed by things that you never even noticed. I have had patients who are very disturbed by the changes that are taking place because they're shocked by the fierceness of their irritability and the sharpness of their mood swings. In fact, I've had patients with pulse rate twice the normal rate! Wild mood swings and increased irritability are linked to the sudden shifts in hormonal balance. These fluctuations in the levels of oestrogen, testosterone, and progesterone can occur when your body doesn't get the right kind of support to maintain natural balance. Sometimes, mood swings can take you high and you feel intense joy in everything around you—a movie or a dish you ordered for dinner. Other times, however, they can take you on a roller-coaster ride of emotions such as sadness, anger, despair, anxiety, or fear.

A MENTAL SHIFT

The 40s are also a time when many women find that they are at the peak of their career and this comes with added expectations and pressure. While the 20s were spent trying to climb the ladder of success, the 30s were about consolidating your presence in the workplace. But it's in your 40s, when you have the experience to back your ideas and with the financial strength that you command, that it all comes together for you.

For homemakers too, this is the time when they assert their independence. By this age, a woman realizes that time has passed her by and that she now has to make some changes in her life—to do things her way. Many women show a lot more independence now than they ever did in their lives. When they were younger, they were dependant on their husband or parents. There's also the feeling that they couldn't do much to change their situation because the kids were too young. So if women are not happy in their relationships, this is the time that they assert themselves.

But that assertiveness can have a dark side too. I've noticed that for certain women, this phase brings out a side of their personality that was dormant for several years. Let me give you an example. My husband and I have been friends with a married couple for many years now. They had a love marriage and now have two children who are in their teens. Ever since we've known them, this couple has been very happy. But about three to four years ago, things started to change. I noticed a change in the attitude of the wife. A woman who for so long was happy to just be known as someone's wife, suddenly was coming into her own. She was a lot more confident and extremely focused on her looks. Whenever the two of us would meet for lunch, she'd only talk about how it was important to be your own person and that now she was keen to do things her own way. She had always been slightly plump, but now she was an active member at her gym and exercised regularly. She had become a completely different person from the one I had known for so many years. I was glad that she was happy with the changes she had made in her life, but was also taken aback by the aggression behind those changes. Soon after, her husband told me that she had been having an affair with a man she met at the gym, and that they had started living separately.

What I realized then was that lakhs of women, after years and years of making adjustments to live according to how their husbands and in-laws want them to, realize that there's more to life as they get older. The realization that the person they have moulded themselves to be is not what they started out as can be very crushing. And that's when they start to rebel because they don't want to be that person anymore. One of the main reasons for this is that women in their 40s often have a lot of free time at hand and don't know what to do with it. If you aren't a working woman, you don't have many positives in your life at this stage. I call that a 'vacuum'. So the woman either goes on a downward spiral and becomes depressed, or she becomes like my friend—rebels and starts to live life on her own terms.

The woman has to deal with herself for the first time in her adult life. That's probably why, as I have observed, a lot of couples experience trouble in their marriage in their 40s. Whether you divorce or not depends on what your social environment allows you to do. I always encourage women to work. At 25, if you aren't a working woman, you don't realize that you may feel empty when you are older. Starting work at 40, when you have no skills or experience, is not easy! This is also the time when women try to reclaim old friends. Indian women tend to lose touch with their school friends after they get married. But suddenly, in the mid-40s, the friends start reconnecting because all of them have time on their hands. So now, a woman has a social circle of her own that's not dependant on her husband. A lot of times, the parents of her children's friends, or neighbours her age, become her friends. As anthropologist Margaret Mead said, 'There is no greater power in the world than the zest of a menopausal woman.'

The symptoms you feel through perimenopause will ultimately influence your actions and reactions. Don't let these symptoms define you during this stage of your life. The power to help yourself during this time lies with the best person—you.

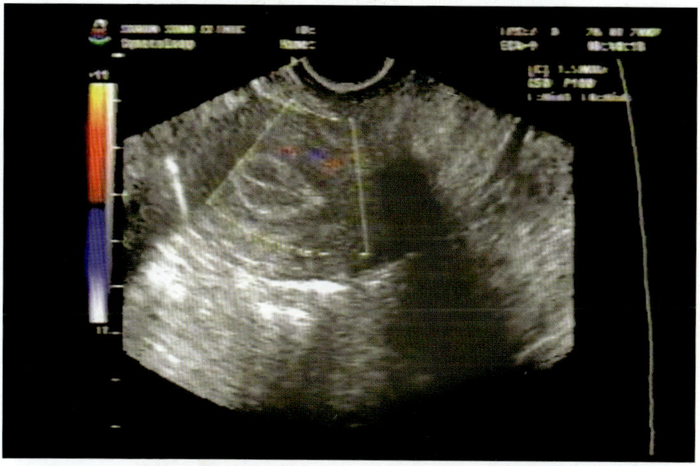

Fig. 1 Sonography picture of the uterus and endometrium

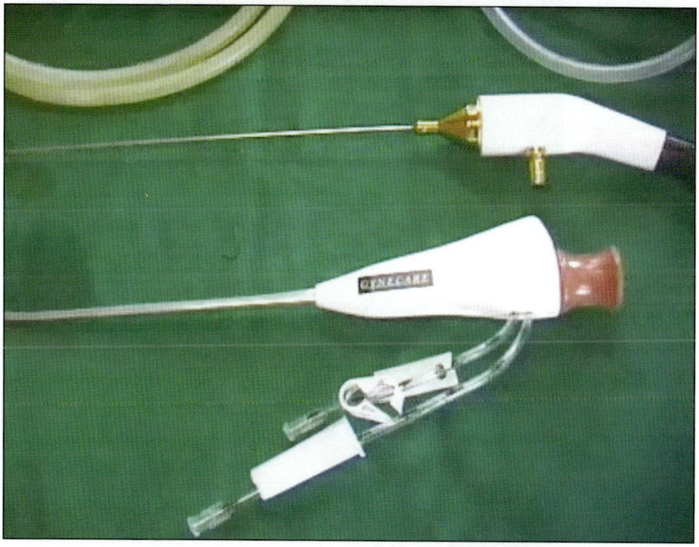

Fig. 2 Thin hysteroscope for office hysteroscopy

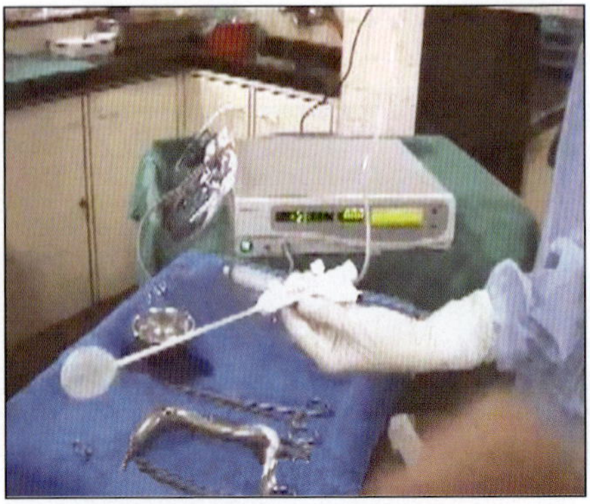

Fig. 3 Balloon ablation for heavy bleeding

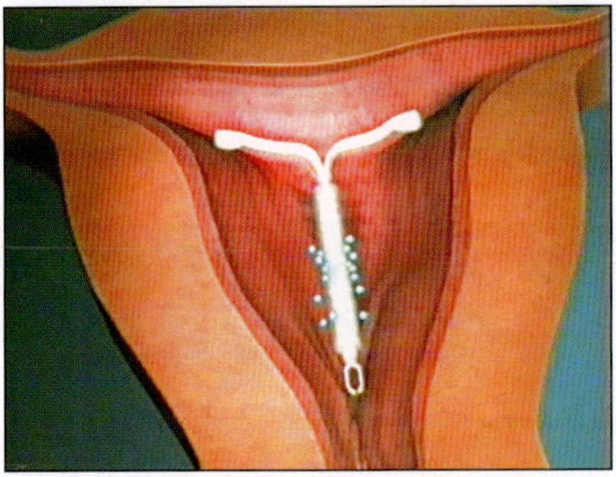

Fig. 4 Hormone intra uterine device-Mirena

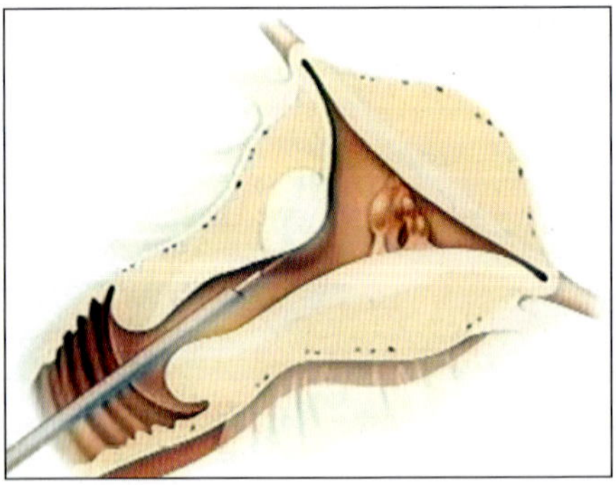

Fig. 5 Versapoint hysteroscopy surgery for submucous fibroid

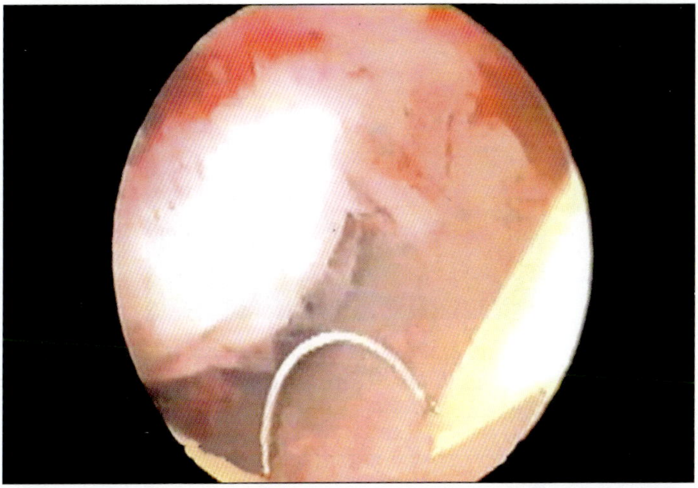

Fig. 6 Submucous fibroid-Removal with hysteroscopic surgery

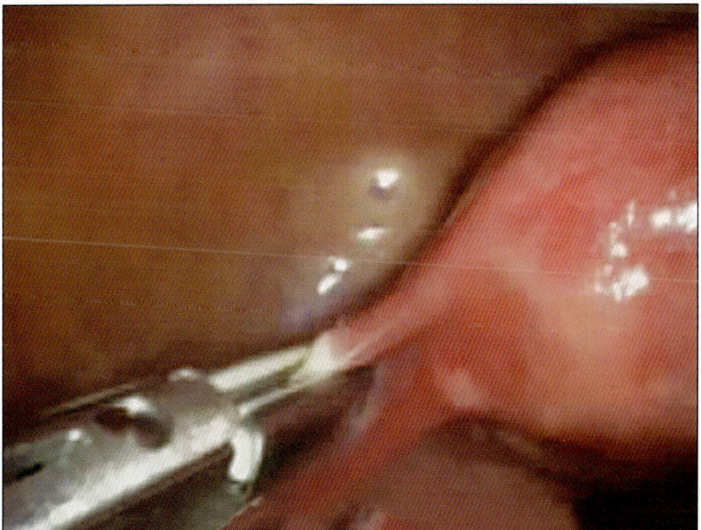

Fig. 7 Uterus removal by laparoscopy

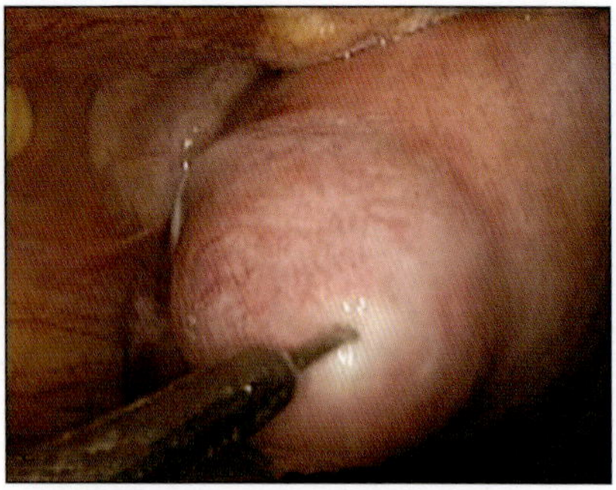

Fig. 8 Serosal fibroid-Removal with laparoscopic surgery

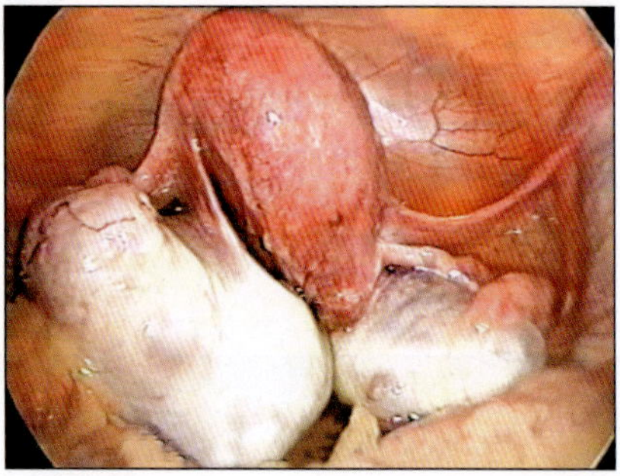

Fig. 9 Ovarian endometrioma

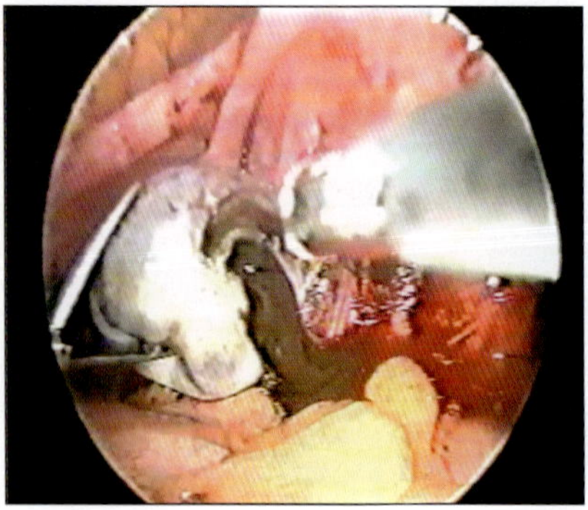

Fig. 10 Endometriotic cyst being operated

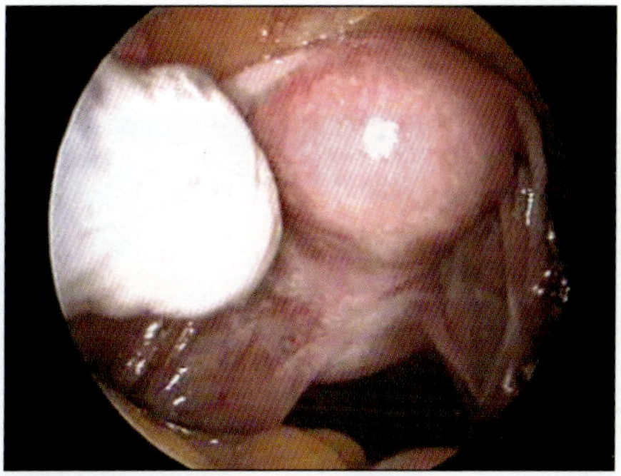

Fig. 11 Laparoscopic image of uterus, ovary, and tubes

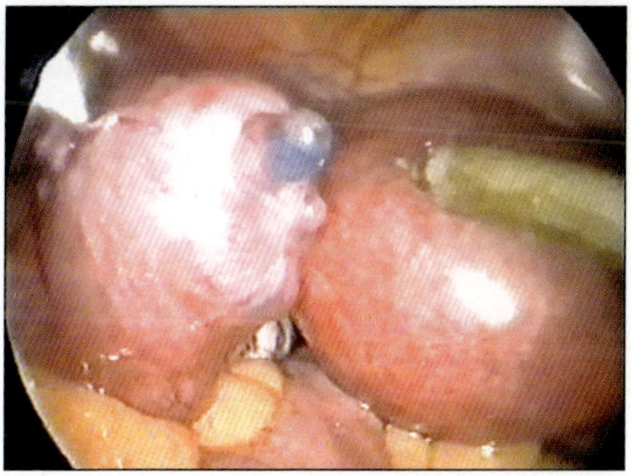

Fig. 12 Tubal block hydrosalpinx

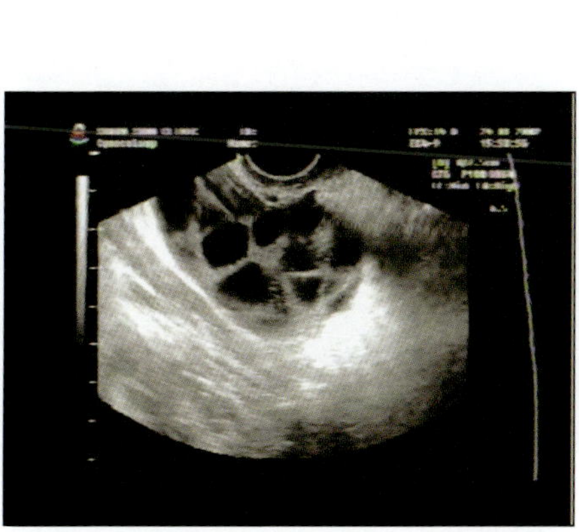

Fig. 13 Polycystic ovary after stimulation

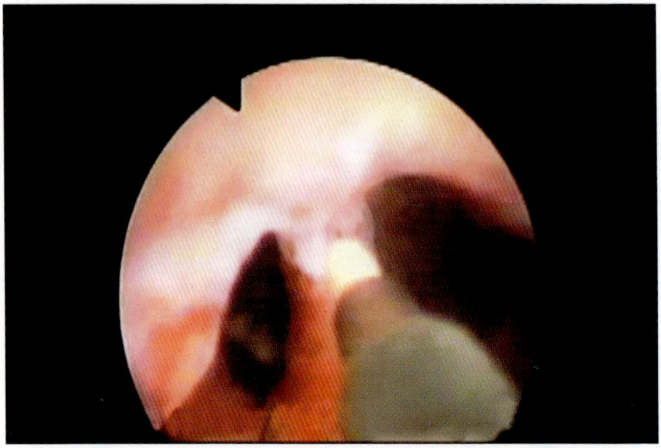

Fig. 14 Septum in uterus-hysteroscopic removal

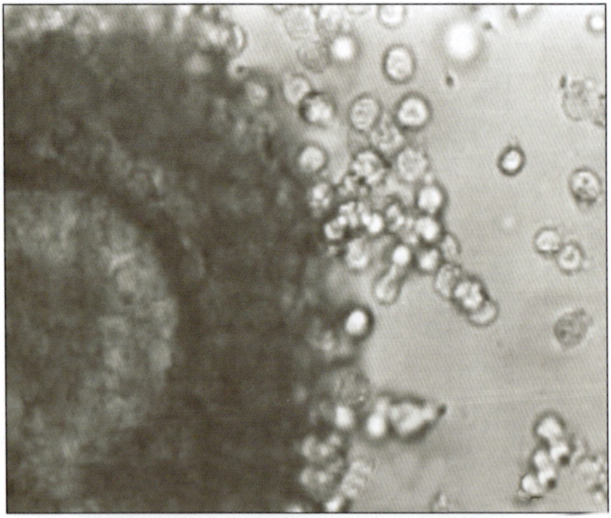

Fig. 15 In-vitro Fertilization (IVF)

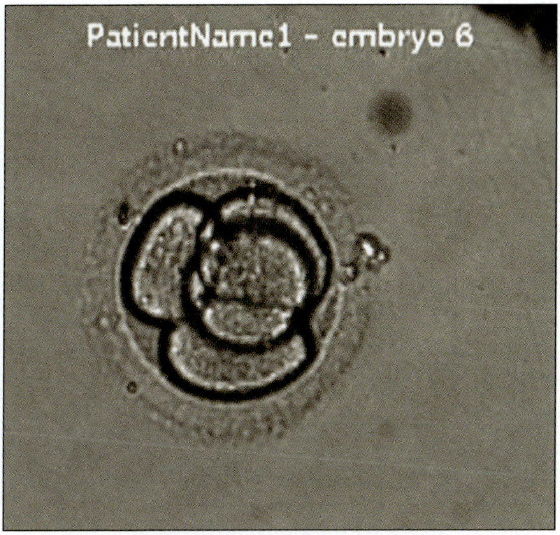

Fig. 16 Embryoscope image of the embryo

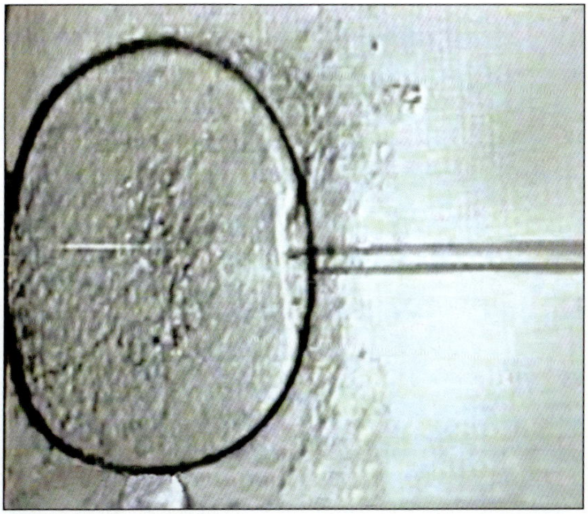

Fig. 17 Intracytoplasmic Sperm Injection (ICSI)

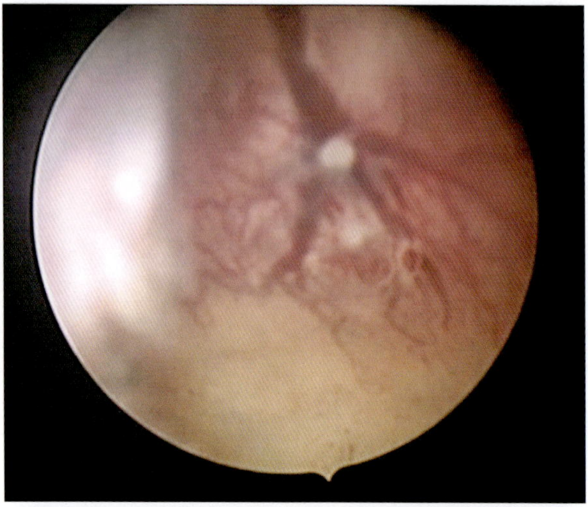

Fig. 18 Endometrial carcinoma

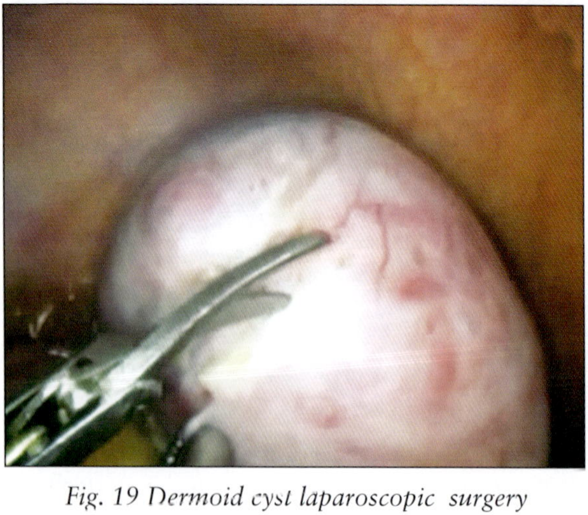

Fig. 19 Dermoid cyst laparoscopic surgery

Part 2

Feeling 40

'I have gratitude. I know myself better. I feel more capable than ever. And as far as the physicality of it, I feel better at 40 than I did at 25.'

— Cameron Diaz

GYNAECOLOGICAL PROBLEMS OCCUR IN ALL women. But as you grow older, they become more serious and could go on to have long-term effects. Many gynaecological problems lack obvious symptoms and can hence remain undetected. If left untreated, they can further weaken your 40-year-old body. Let's take a look at a few gynaecological conditions that affect women after they cross 40.

4

Bleeding

Menstrual disorders are one of the most common complaints that women in this part of the menopausal transition experience. Bleeding is a major problem of the 40s. Even women who've always have regular periods will have bleeding issues in their 40s. The irregularity in the period and the change in quantity is what brings on the changes. Some women may have a lot of bleeding, while others, scanty. And, of course, there are woman who've had a problem with their periods for a long time, maybe because of hormonal problems like polycystic ovarian syndrome or conditions such as fibroids etc., and the problem just continues into their 40s.

Before we try to understand why women in their 40s have this problem, here are the different terms your doctor might use when talking about bleeding related problems.

Menorrahagia: Abnormally heavy periods at regular intervals that lasts more than 7 days.
Metrorrhagia: Flow at irregular intervals.
Menometrorrhagia: Frequent and excessive blood flow.
Polymenorrhoea: Bleeding at intervals of less than 21 days.
Dysmenorrhoea: Experiencing pain during menstruation.

So, how do you know if you have heavy bleeding? Heavy bleeding occurs when you need to change your tampon or sanitary pad after less than two hours or you pass large clots. Women over 40 years of age who are still menstruating can get an increase in bleeding severity due to a final squeeze of oestrogen as the body prepares itself for the approaching menopause.

In order to discuss irregular periods, let's first understand what a normal period is. While every woman is different, normal periods have an interval of 25 to 31 days from the beginning of one period to another, with bleeding lasting around 5 days. For instance, when a woman has her period on the 1st of the month, she only ovulates on the 14th and she'll get her next period on the 28th. This is how the menstrual cycle usually takes place. A woman releases oestrogen in response to pituitary hormones in the first half of the cycle. After ovulation, progesterone is also produced. Oestrogen and progesterone help prepare the lining of the uterus—also called the endometrium—with a thick layer to receive a fertilized egg. These hormones peak approximately 7–10 days after ovulation. In the absence of a pregnancy, the lining sheds. Thus, a period takes place and the cycle will then repeat.

Abnormal uterine bleeding includes:

- Periods that are too frequent, more often than every 26 days.
- Heavy periods, with passage of large clots.
- Bleeding at the wrong time, including spotting or pink-tinged vaginal discharge.
- Bleeding lasting longer than 7 days.
- Extremely light periods or no periods at all.

One of the common reasons for irregular heavy bleeding is anovulation. In this condition the egg is not released from the ovary every month, like it usually does. So the regular ovulation that used to happen monthly doesn't happen anymore. It is common in perimenopausal woman.

It doesn't mean that a 45-year-old woman does not ovulate. It means that she may not ovulate regularly—maybe once in two or three months. And because you don't get your period if you don't ovulate, it becomes less frequent. If your period doesn't come one month, the ovaries still produce oestrogen. But the egg doesn't rupture, so the progesterone is not formed. This means the lining of the uterus will become thicker and thicker. So a lot of women have oestrogenic bleeding only. And if the period has not come for two months, the lining cannot be sustained because it's too thick, resulting in heavy bleeding. This is not controlled bleeding because it's not balanced with the progesterone, which is also responsible for controlling the intensity and duration of menstrual bleeding. Blood loss during heavy bleeding can be so severe that it can cause a dangerously lowered blood count, also known as anaemia, which can lead to medical complications and symptoms such as dizziness and fainting.

This is what happens when a woman suffers from anovulation. That's why the period goes on for more than the usual five days because of the absence of the balancing hormone, progesterone. Remember, this is not a pathological problem because she has no disease. This is a strictly hormonal problem, but can still lead to cancer of the uterus if uncontrolled for a long time. That is why it is important to have regular periods—a 25 to 35 day cycle is perfect.

When a 45-year-old woman comes to me with heavy bleeding, after examining her, I first do a sonography test. (See Fig. 1 in the insert pages.) In many cases, the test shows that the woman's uterus lining is very thick. As thick endometrium takes a long time to come out, she bleeds longer and heavier. Though not common, menorrhagia can be a sign of endometrial cancer. A potentially precancerous condition, known as endometrial hyperplasia, can also result in abnormal vaginal bleeding. This situation is more frequent in women who are over the age of 40. That's when we do a biopsy. If we find that she has simple endometrial hyperplasia, it's easily reversible with drugs. We give her progesterone for 10–12 days every month to stabilize the endometrium and get her menstrual cycle back on track.

But sometimes the situation advances to complex hyperplasia. That condition is one step away from cancer. I have to keep a very careful watch on patients going through this condition. It can be controlled with hormonal medication and careful monitoring or sometimes removal of the uterus is a better option. Irregular, heavy, and continuous periods at this age cannot be neglected. A lot of women neglect it because they think they are undergoing menopause and that this is a normal part of it. That's why a lot of women don't do anything about the changes happening in their bodies unless they are suffering really badly or what they're undergoing is radically different from what their friends are experiencing. So they learn to live with it. But it's not necessary that you suffer so much even before you start menopause.

HOW DO YOU DETECT THE PROBLEM?

The first step is to review the history of symptoms and menstrual periods. The gynaecologist will determine whether you are ovulating regularly using:

- Your menstrual calendar.
- A pelvic examination.
- A progesterone test. Low levels during the third week of your menstrual cycle suggest an ovulation problem.
- An endometrial biopsy during the fourth week of your menstrual cycle. Perimenopausal women typically have an endometrial biopsy because abnormal endometrial tissue is common in this age group.

- A transvaginal pelvic ultrasound to check for abnormalities in the pelvic area. It helps diagnose the cause of abnormal bleeding. If a pelvic mass is found, ultrasound results are useful for making treatment decisions.

If your symptoms are severe, these blood tests are ordered:

- Pregnancy test (human chorionic gonadotropin, or hCG).
- Complete blood count to check for signs of disease, infection, and anaemia.
- Thyroid-stimulating hormone to check for a thyroid gland problem, which can cause irregular periods.
- Serum prolactin level to check for a pituitary gland problem, which can interfere with or stop your menstrual cycle.
- Serum ferritin to check for anaemia, a symptom of heavy blood loss.
- Urine test to screen for infection or disease.
- Pap smear and cultures to check for infection or abnormal cervical cells.
- Endometrial biopsy, usually for the perimenopausal woman, to learn whether the endometrium is healthy and functioning normally.
- Hysteroscopy, which involves inserting a thin pencil like camera into the womb, to check for and treat a suspected condition such as uterine fibroids or if bleeding continues despite treatment. (See Fig. 2 in the insert pages.)

HOW DO WE FIGHT IT?

There are many solutions to heavy bleeding ranging from simple to the radical. Bleeding in the perimenopause is often abnormal uterine bleeding (AUB), also called dysfunctional uterine bleeding (DUB), where there is no obvious cause found . Since these are normally hormonal problems, we can solve them by hormonal therapy. Most women are scared of hormonal therapy because they believe it'll cause cancer. But fresh guidance from the British Menopause Society says that the benefits of HRT outweigh any potential risk for women.[1]

The simplest solution we have is to put the patient on birth-control pills. They contain hormones that can stop the lining of your uterus from getting too thick. They can also help keep your menstrual cycle regular and reduce cramping.

There are also treatments which I call '10 minute solutions to heavy bleeding'.

One of these simple treatments is the uterine balloon ablation therapy. (See Fig. 3 in the insert pages.) This involves putting a small tube with an attached inflatable balloon at the top, into the womb through the vagina. This doesn't involve any cuts or stitches. The balloon is filled with hot water at 87°C through a computerized machine, and the lining of the womb is heated for 8 minutes. The balloon catheter is then removed and discarded. This high temperature burns and thins the lining of the womb and prevents it from growing. This procedure can be done under local or general anaesthesia and can be safely done even in patients who have medical problems such as diabetes, high blood pressure, heart or kidney disease, where other operations are risky to perform. This results either in stoppage or reduction in menstrual bleeding permanently. The patient needs to be in the hospital only for a few hours and is fit to resume work from the next day. This is a permanent procedure where without removing the uterus and without any surgery, in a few minutes, we can completely solve the problem of heavy bleeding.

Another solution is TCRE (Transcervical Resection of the Endometrium) where a telescope with a camera is put inside the uterus and the entire lining of the uterus is shaved off using a blade like device with electric current in it. This again takes about 30 minutes and the woman's period can be stopped permanently without needing to do a major surgery.

The other simple, non-surgical method of treating heavy bleeding is to insert a hormonal intrauterine device, called the levonorgestrel (LNg) intrauterine device (IUD). This is a small T-shaped device, which looks like a Copper-T or a loop, but has hormones inside it. This can be placed inside the uterus in two minutes, without any anaesthesia, and once inside the womb, the hormones that are released, reduce or stop bleeding during menstruation for five years. It has the added benefit of contraception. This is a temporary method and the device can be removed at any time in a minute in the gynaecologist's office. (See Fig. 4 in the insert pages.)

Many women with heavy bleeding decide to undergo removal of the uterus (hysterectomy) as a permanent solution to their problem and many gynaecologists encourage it. This may be too radical a treatment for DUB. However, there are plenty of women who believe that once the uterus is removed, they may put on weight. That is just not true. What happens is that women rest for about six months after the hysterectomy even though it is absolutely not required, and the lack of exercise is what enables the weight gain. Also, many women have a mental block to the removal of the womb as they feel they may lose their femininity or sexual appetite. Thus, the emphasis is on simple alternatives to hysterectomy because not everyone wants to undergo uterus removal surgery.

5

Fibroids

Hormonal issues aren't the only reason for heavy periods. There are other issues as well. One of the most common problems is that of fibroids. While women in their 30s also suffer from fibroids, they are also common in the 40s. Fibroids are simple tumours that form inside the uterus; they are usually not cancerous.

Around 30 percent of women suffer from fibroids. It is not known why fibroids develop, but their growth, though not necessarily their cause, is related to oestrogen. Several things suggest their dependence on hormones: Fibroids rarely grow in girls before puberty; pregnancy can spur their growth, and they often shrink after menopause. They can cause bleeding problems, pain, infertility, and recurrent miscarriages, depending on their location and their size. If they're pressing up against the urinary bladder, they can cause urinary problems; if they are pressing against the rectum, they can lead to problems in passing stool. Many women are unaware that they have fibroids, as the symptoms are not very obvious.

How big can they get?

The uterus is usually 7cm long—the size of your fist. Some fibroids are as small as a pebble. Others can grow large and multiply in number, causing a woman's abdomen to become enlarged. I have removed fibroids that are 14cm—that's double the size of the uterus! Doctors measure the size of fibroids in pregnancy terms. So a 20-week fibroid is as big as the uterus would be in the fifth month of a woman's pregnancy. Larger fibroids can take up too much space in the pelvis and press against surrounding organs, including the bladder and colon, which can lead to frequent urination and constipation. Fibroids may also interfere with fertility. But the biggest complaint about these benign growths is the heavy bleeding that can make a woman a virtual prisoner in her home during her periods. A routine pelvic exam initially can detect the presence of fibroids, and they can be confirmed by procedures like sonography or MRI scans.

Is hysterectomy a solution?

Fibroids are, unfortunately, recurrent tumours. Even when you treat a woman in her 30s and remove all her fibroids, they are very likely to come back when she's in her 40s. These are estrogen dependent tumours, so as long as the woman has hormones in her body, the fibroids will continue to grow.

These days, most fibroids are removed laproscopically using keyhole surgery. Fibroids that cause bleeding problems are found on the inner lining of the uterus. Those can be reached by hysteroscopy. For younger women who want to have children in the future, we go through the vagina with a thin telescope with a camera attached to it into the uterus and shave off the fibroid using a blade with an electric current (resectoscope), or a laser like device (versapoint). (See Fig. 5 in the insert pages.) But in the 40s, if the woman is done planning her family, and if we've already removed fibroids from her when she was younger, doctors usually recommend that the uterus be removed. That's because a hysterectomy is the only way you can ensure fibroids don't return. (See Fig. 6 in the insert pages.) The uterus can be removed laproscopically, or through the vagina, or via open surgery if the problem is of a more serious nature. (See Fig. 7 in the insert pages.) Personally, my clinical practice has shown that most patients don't want to have a hysterectomy.

I have a friend in her late 40s who, about five years ago, was suffering from multiple fibroids. She insisted that she did not want a hysterectomy. Normally, most doctors recommend opting for a hysterectomy if the patient has heavy bleeding and fibroids because even if you remove the fibroids, the bleeding problem could continue due to abnormal hormones in the perimenopause. But my friend did not want that and we removed 13 fibroids from her using laparoscopic surgery. She went into natural menopause a couple of years later, so the uterus wasn't of much use to her in that sense. But psychologically, it was important to her that the uterus be present in her body. After that incident, I realized that even gynaecologists are insensitive to the psychological impact of a hysterectomy. There are a lot of scandals about women having their uterus removed when they are young because some doctors remove the uterus even for the smallest of problems once the woman has completed her family. There is very little sensitivity among doctors about the importance of the uterus to a woman. I am personally not very fond of removing the uterus. Just because a particular organ is not required doesn't mean that we remove it. As long as it's not diseased, we should try and keep the organ.

Interestingly, hysterectomy comes from the word 'hysteria' and women have always had a lot of apprehension about undergoing that surgery. There was a strong belief a few decades ago that removing the uterus would make a woman hysterical. So it still has a psychological bearing on women. I have patients who ask me if a hysterectomy will affect their mind. I've heard that question many times, but it never fails to surprise me. Women don't understand that the uterus is like the appendix. It is of no use once you have had children. Several women believe that their sexuality will be affected if they have their uterus removed; that they will now be less of a woman and it'll affect their relationship with their husbands. But that's not true. If you're worried that your sex drive might be less than it was before your hysterectomy, or that your partner might not find you as appealing, talk with other women who have had a hysterectomy. You may be surprised to learn that they still enjoy an active and satisfying sex life. Having said that, a hysterectomy could have side-effects because we still don't know everything about the human body and how it'll react to certain situations. While each woman who has a hysterectomy may have a unique reaction, there are many changes in the body that are typical among most women. If your ovaries are removed along with your uterus, you may experience hot flashes or other menopause symptoms. But if the ovaries are conserved, there are no hormonal changes in the body as the uterus contains no hormones. Another important factor to consider is your age. Your potential emotional reaction to hysterectomy is often age-related. Generally, the older you are when you have it done, the less emotional you are likely to get about it.

SO WHAT ARE THE OTHER OPTIONS?

You have to understand that just because there's a uterine fibroid doesn't mean that you have to operate on it. If it's not causing problems, you can leave it alone. Although fibroids aren't life-threatening, their symptoms can drastically alter a woman's quality of life. If the fibroid is on the inner lining, it is called a submucous fibroid. It has to be removed through hysteroscopy and then shaved off. This can be done using a machine called resectoscope or the new technique using the versapoint. The versapoint is a laser-like device with which the fibroid can be vapourized. This is a safe and very simple procedure and you can even go home that same day. Fibroids that are large and are located on the outer side of the uterus (intramural or serosal) are removed laproscopically or through open surgery by making a cut on the abdominal wall. Keep in mind that there is no effective medical treatment for fibroids. So be careful of quacks and 'well-meaning' friends who recommend pills or alternative medicines to treat fibroids.

One of the common treatments that a lot of gynaecologists employ is to induce temporary menopause for between six months and a year with the help of medicines and injections. The injections suppress oestrogen production. When the patient doesn't produce any hormones, the fibroids will not grow. She will not have her menstrual period or any pain related to it. The reason we do this is to increase the patient's haemoglobin level. I've had patients who bleed heavily and are scared of surgery. A couple of my patients had haemoglobin of 4 and 5 and severe weakness. And they were living their everyday life with that little haemoglobin in their body. For such women, it makes sense to induce temporary menopause so that they can build up their haemoglobin. That's better than giving 4–5 units of blood since you can't operate on a woman whose haemoglobin is that low. They are given iron capsules to build up their blood, and as they won't have their period, they will not lose more blood. We then remove the fibroids and in a few months, they are off menopause and hopefully, things are back to normal. But it's important to know that this treatment cannot be used as contraception. So thankfully, they do not affect a woman's fertility when she stops taking treatment.

Two years ago, a new treatment to remove fibroids was introduced. It's called MRI-guided Focussed Ultrasound. Here, the woman has to lie in the MRI machine, just like she would for a normal MRI test. On the machine, there are ultrasound rays that pass through her abdominal wall to the fibroid. The beam is focussed onto the area of the fibroid. The imaging and treatment is controlled on a computer in another room. The rays burn the fibroid millimetre by millimetre. This technique usually takes between one to two hours. Over a period of time, the fibroid shrinks. Patients who have a high-risk for surgery or those who are scared to undergo an operation can now walk in, treat their fibroids, and walk out without an operation. The uterus is preserved and so is fertility. The procedure has a very low-risk of complications and hence is a simple, safe, and effective treatment for fibroids. For women who've had to have repeated surgery for the removal of fibroids, this is a wonderful option.

Subserosal fibroids are those which grow on the outer side of the uterus. These usually cause no problems unless they grow very big and the patient begins to experience difficulty in passing urine or stools. They can be removed by the old method of making a cut on the abdomen, opening the abdomen, and removing the tumour. Later, the gap in the womb is stitched and the abdomen is closed. This method requires longer hospitalization and the recovery period is also longer. Nowadays, most of the fibroids can be removed by keyhole (laparoscopic) surgery. By this method, a telescope is put into the stomach through a very small cut on the stomach wall. This telescope has a camera attached to it and the entire operation is done by watching it on a TV screen. The surgery is cosmetic as there is no large scar. Also, the patient has to stay in hospital only for 2–3 days and has less pain. (See Fig. 8 in the insert pages.)

Intramural fibroids lie in the middle of the womb and may cause pain during periods and sometimes problems during pregnancy if they are large. These fibroids may prevent a normal delivery or cause heavy bleeding or infection after delivery.

Since fibroids may be found in women of all ages from those in their 20s to those in their 50s, it is good for all women to have regular gynaecological check-ups even if they have no symptoms.

Fibroids are three times more common in black women than any other race. That's why I wasn't surprised when I removed 55 fibroids from an African patient who was in her late 30s. I can't even imagine the pain she must have lived with because of so many fibroids. Normally, if the situation is so grave, I immediately suggest a hysterectomy. But that wasn't an option because she was keen on having children.

She was an infertility patient and had multiple surgeries before she came to me. By the time we both finally met, her uterus was already 28 weeks pregnancy size because of the fibroids. That's like being in your seventh month of pregnancy. She even looked pregnant. We had to have an open surgery because the fibroids were too big to have been removed laproscopically. She had fibroids of all sizes—small, medium, and large. I kept on removing them and realized at the end of it that we had removed 55 fibroids! This was a very unusual surgery for me. After the surgery, her uterus did not look healthy enough for her to have a baby. But in the next three months, there was considerable recovery and the uterus looked a lot healthier.

Another patient of mine had a 24-week sized uterus. She had already had an embolization due to a large fibroid, which is a non-surgical way of treating fibroids by blocking off the arteries that feed the fibroids, the uterine arteries, and making the fibroids shrink. This reduced the size of the fibroid and made it less likely to bleed during surgery. She then underwent a major open surgery to remove the fibroid in a small town, and during this, the uterus was badly damaged. But she was still unable to have a baby and that's when she came to me for a solution. I advised her to not to have a baby because her uterus was very scarred and there was a high-risk of its rupturing during pregnancy. So we opted for IVF with surrogacy for her and her surrogate is now pregnant. Her eggs were removed and fertilized with her husband's sperms and the baby was created. But as her uterus was damaged we implanted the baby in the surrogate's womb. This way she has her baby and there is no serious risk to her health.

6

Prolapse

Prolapse literally means 'to fall' or 'slip out of place', and in a woman's body, it relates to the uterus, urinary bladder, and rectum. There are many causes for prolapse, but the two main causes, gravity and childbirth, can affect us all. So it's important that you keep an eye out for symptoms. Prolapse can be fairly mild but it can also become serious, and once the damage is done, it is virtually impossible to undo it.

The uterus, bladder, and rectum are supported by a hammock of muscles slung between the tailbone and the pubic bone. These muscles are known as the pelvic floor muscles. Ligaments and connective tissues also anchor the uterus in place. If these tissues are weakened or damaged, the uterus can slip down into the vagina.

This is called prolapse—looseness or descent of the genital organs. Prolapse of the uterus is common around menopause because the muscle support often becomes thinner when the hormone levels, in particular oestrogen, are reduced.

Prolapse can actually happen at any age. Nulliparous prolapse happens to women who have never had a baby and this is due to an inherent genetic weakness of the supporting tissues. But this is an extremely rare condition. The more common type of prolapse is in parous women—where a woman who had given birth and, in her later age is suffering from prolapse.

What the patient typically comes with is complaints of something coming out of the vagina. That, however, is a more serious degree of prolapse. It usually starts with looseness of the vagina. It's either the woman who will realize the laxity during sex, as she doesn't feel the same sensations as she did before childbirth and delivery, or her husband will point it out. In the first stage, there's just general vaginal looseness or mild leakage of urine. In the second degree, part of the genital organs, like the uterus, will start coming out of the vagina. Every time the uterus comes out, it drags along with it the bladder and the rectum. The urinary bladder also almost always descends along with the uterus and the rectum as well. That's because these are all closely connected, almost touching, in the pelvic region. In the third stage, the uterus is literally lying outside the vagina. Lots and lots of women walk around with the entire uterus out of the body. They live with it as a way of life and push it back in at regular intervals. They usually wear a tight pad to keep it in place even though it causes discomfort while walking. But that is an extreme degree of prolapse. Instances like this are more in our country because the Indian women somehow have the capacity to tolerate a lot.

Prolapse is more common among women from the slightly lower social strata since they are likely to have more number of natural deliveries. Also, the strength and tone of your pelvic muscles and ligaments depends a lot on the right nutrition. So any trauma, injury, or stress to that area would result in prolapse when the woman gets older. And when normal deliveries or forcep deliveries are not conducted very carefully, the risk of prolapse is much higher. But that's not to say that women from the higher social strata don't suffer from prolapse because it depends on the inherent strength of your pelvis support. In the higher social strata, newborn babies are normally bigger. For example, if you have a 3.5 kilo baby, you are much more likely to have injury to the vagina and pelvic support during delivery than when you deliver a 2 kilo baby. Prolapse is typically seen in women who've had normal delivery. Those who've had a C-section have almost no trauma to the passage, and so they rarely suffer from prolapse. Their vaginas are very likely to be the same as when they didn't have any children. Even a single normal delivery increases your chances of prolapse. If it is a long labour, where the head is constantly pounding on the pelvic support, it could mean you'll suffer from prolapse in your 40s.

The uterus is located in the pelvis, in the middle of a hammock like support. If this support loosens or tears, the organs tend to slide down. Everything gets stretched and it doesn't snap back into position. So a prolonged, difficult delivery, a huge baby, the use of forceps, any vaginal tear, the mother's nutrition status, the genetic strength of the ligaments—all of these contribute to a woman's chances of suffering from prolapse.

Severe coughing associated with conditions such as chronic bronchitis or asthma and constipation where there is chronic straining to empty the bowel can also cause prolapse. Some women also suffer from prolapse immediately after delivery, but it's not that common. By the time a woman is in her late 30, she starts to notice stress urinary incontinence and laxity of the vagina during intercourse. Almost every woman who's had a normal delivery will have an element of prolapse, though it may be so mild as to be irrelevant.

WHAT CAN WE DO ABOUT IT?

We examine such patients and first determine the stage of prolapse. Depending on the level of discomfort the patent is experiencing and how much it's affecting her lifestyle, we advise the necessary treatment. A lot of times when the organ comes out of the body, there is friction and irritation because it rubs against the thighs, causing ulceration in the area. The ulcerated area can become infected and ooze pus. The area of that organ that's rubbing against the thighs becomes thicker and hard. Continuous or uncontrolled urine discharge is also common.

There are a lot of conservative surgeries for prolapse. With a younger 40-year-old patient, for example, we can take the vaginal approach, and from the vagina, cut off the excess tissues that have formed. We then reposition the uterus and tighten the bladder and the rectum. With a laparoscopy or with a small bikini cut, we can pull the uterus up and put it in place with a tape. Using the woman's own tissues is not possible because they've become very weak. These are called sling operations.

Sometimes special mesh is used to strengthen the ligaments where they are weak or torn. As the body heals, the mesh helps form stronger tissues to give more support where it is needed. In women who are older and who are comfortable with the removal of the uterus, more often than not, a vaginal hysterectomy is done. That's because the uterus has come down so much that it's just easier to remove it from there. Unfortunately, even with a vaginal hysterectomy, as the woman grows older, there are chances of the vaginal wall collapsing. The vagina is like a tunnel that also starts to collapse because the tissues have become weaker, paper-thin, and have lost their elasticity. This is called a vault prolapse. That is pretty difficult to repair and we use a laparoscopic approach to take the vagina up and fix it.

CAN YOU LIVE WITH IT?

Prolapse doesn't hurt, which is why women tend to live with it. If it was painful, they would've visited the doctor at the first signs of discomfort. A lot of women make do with wearing a sanitary pad 24x7 because even if you leak urine, the pad will absorb it. Women suffering from prolapse can even have sex. You can push the organ back and continue with normal sexual activities. Couples manage, probably because they are scared of surgery or are embarrassed about it.

I have a friend who from the looks of it was doing very well. She was always the first one to hit the dance floor at parties. You wouldn't think there was anything wrong with her because she acted so normally around us. She didn't tell us about it for a long time, but one day she said that she was suffering from third degree prolapse. Her entire uterus was coming out of her vagina. And she used to wear something to keep it in place because it was just hanging between her legs. It was hindering her everyday activities and she was doing everything she could to push the uterus back and hold it in place. Even though she had access to a gynaecologist friend in me, she was embarrassed to discuss this problem. So I can only imagine how many women out there must be suffering silently, not sharing this with anyone or going to a doctor. This was quite an eye-opener for me and should be one for you as well. Remember, prolapse is nothing to be embarrassed about. It's better to get it treated than suffer silently for years.

WHAT CAN BE DONE TO PREVENT PROLAPSE?

As with most things, it is much better to prevent prolapse than try to fix it. Women who are overweight are at a greater risk of prolapse. As prolapse happens due to weak pelvic tissues and pelvic floor muscles, all women should keep their pelvic floor muscles strong, no matter what their age. Pelvic floor muscles, just like any other muscles, can be made stronger with the right exercises. Sample exercises are given on page 79.

But these exercises need to be done correctly and practiced long enough to strengthen the muscles. Ask your gynaecologist to suggest a physiotherapist. Learn what causes prolapse and make necessary lifestyle changes, such as improving your diet, fluid intake, exercising, and losing weight. It can help you deal with it better. It also helps to be aware of good bowel and bladder habits to avoid straining. Make sure your delivery is conducted by experts so the risk of tears and injuries to the vagina and perineum are less. If your gynaecologist advises a caesarian section due to a comparatively large baby or possible difficult delivery, discuss it with the doctor properly and make an informed choice, not just irrationally insist on trying for a normal delivery.

Another non-surgical solution is to insert a pessary. It is a flexible device which can be fitted into the vagina to support the uterus. There are different shapes and sizes of pessaries. A bangle like rubber ring pessary is freely available in India. You can remove and re-insert the pessary much like a tampon. Vaginal pessaries can be an effective way of reducing the symptoms of a prolapse, but they are not appropriate for everyone. Together with pelvic floor exercises, they provide a non-surgical solution to manage prolapse.

Can a prolapse lead to other problems?

Stress incontinence is a common condition, and is caused by a variety of factors, including those that can lead to prolapse. Many women first experience stress incontinence during pregnancy, when the weight of the baby presses down on the pelvic floor, weakening bladder control. Following birth, the pelvic floor muscles become weak so that even after several months, the woman cannot regain normal bladder control. Common symptoms of stress incontinence include leaking when you cough, laugh, or sneeze; when you are exercising or lifting, having little warning of the need to urinate, which means that you may not reach the toilet in time, and sometimes an increased urgency to urinate. Some women even dribble urine without realizing it. You often suffer from stress incontinence because of associated prolapse.

7

Stress Urinary Incontinence

To know what's wrong with an organ system, we first need to know how it works. The kidneys make urine continuously. A trickle of urine is constantly passing to the bladder through tubes called ureters. The amount of urine you make depends on how much you drink, eat, and sweat. The bladder is where urine is stored. It expands like a balloon as it fills with urine. The outlet for urine—the urethra—is normally kept closed by pelvic floor muscles beneath the bladder that surround and support the urethra. When a certain volume of urine is in the bladder, messages are sent between the brain, the bladder, and the pelvic floor muscles. These tell you how full your bladder is, and tells the muscles to contract or relax at the right time. That's how you become aware that the bladder is getting full. When you go to the toilet to pass urine, the bladder muscles contract, and the urethra and pelvic floor muscles relax to allow urine to flow out.

How often have you coughed or laughed too hard, and experienced a urinary leakage, but were too embarrassed to tell anyone? You're not alone. A common problem for women in the 40s is stress urinary incontinence (SUI). It occurs when an activity, such as coughing or sneezing, causes a small amount of urine to leak out. Simply put, urinary incontinence is the inability to hold urine upon straining. Stress incontinence is the most common type of incontinence suffered by older women. This can, of course, happen to anybody. But it's most common in women who have had one or two deliveries and are in their 40s. It is an extremely common condition in women who've had normal deliveries. As many as 1 in 5 women over the age of 40 have some degree of stress incontinence. This is unfortunate, as many cases can be successfully treated or significantly improved. It is likely that the true number of people affected is much higher. Many people do not tell their doctor about incontinence due to embarrassment. Some people wrongly think that incontinence is a normal part of ageing or that it cannot be treated. It's the most hidden or less talked about condition. Considering that a lot of women suffer from it, very few women talk about it. Even in my clinic, while women are comfortable coming for something as small as white discharge, very few women will primarily come for SUI.

A number of things can contribute to SUI. For instance,

it can result from weak muscles in the pelvic floor or a weak sphincter muscle at the neck of the bladder. A problem with the way the sphincter muscle opens and closes can also result in stress incontinence. Stress incontinence is often caused by physical changes to the body like pregnancy and childbirth, menstruation, menopause, problems with muscles in the bladder and the urethra, and weakened muscles around the bladder. In cases of SUI, the muscles in the pelvis can weaken. This can cause the bladder to drop down into a position that prevents the urethra from closing completely. The result is a leakage of urine.

Along with SUI, women in their 40s suffer from many other urinary issues. If they have the urge, they cannot hold it and just have to go to the bathroom. Some might even pass urine in their underwear because they cannot hold it. They may not even empty their bladder completely. If they've passed urine five minutes ago, they'll want to go again. If you have to go to the bathroom five times in a night, it can have a serious effect on your health because you are not getting enough sleep.

A lot of urinary issues come up in the 40s and they can be very harrowing for a woman. And most women, unfortunately, don't talk about it. Similarly, even infections are very common. Something like a urinary tract infection (UTI) is very common and recurrent, but is still not talked about. So I, as a doctor, first need to distinguish which issue is the patient dealing with. Is she suffering from overflow incontinence (urine filling up and dribbling over)? Or is she suffering from urge incontinence—even if a little bit of urine fills up, the woman runs to the bathroom because she cannot hold it? There are many different types of incontinence. That's why we need to know about the history of the patient to figure out what's happening.

Only a woman's problem

Men suffer from incontinence much less commonly and if it does happen, they are much older, have an enlarged prostate, or suffer from diseases like diabetes or infections or some malformation of the genital area. Of course, the length of the urethra in men is much longer. Women have a very short urethra.

Some women may have an atonic bladder—a large bladder that has become dilated but is not emptying properly. Because the ability to urinate is impaired, the woman experiences a great deal of pain. An atonic bladder keeps distending and doesn't give the signal for contraction. So we have to give the woman medication that will contract the bladder. Women with an atonic bladder sometimes don't realize that it is full and that it is about to leak.

So how do you treat it?

Firstly, I recommend strengthening the pelvic floor muscles with exercises. About 6 in 10 cases of stress incontinence can be improved with the right exercises. It is important that you exercise the correct muscles. Sit in a chair with your knees slightly apart. Now imagine that you are passing urine and are trying to stop the stream. These are the muscles to strengthen.

Here's how you can do the exercises:

- Sit, stand, or lie with your knees slightly apart. Slowly tighten your pelvic floor muscles under the bladder as hard as you can. Hold till the count of five, then relax. Repeat at least five times. These are called slow pull-ups.
- Then do the same exercise quickly for a second or two. Repeat at least five times. These are called fast pull-ups.
- Keep repeating five slow pull-ups and five fast pull-ups for five minutes.

Aim to do these exercises for about five minutes at least three times a day. If you are overweight and lack control of your excretory functions, you should first try to lose weight. Surgery is an option if the problem continues. If you do regular pelvic floor exercises during pregnancy and after you have the baby, then stress incontinence is less likely to develop following childbirth and later in life.

Some incontinence problems have to be treated medically with long-term use of daily medication. There are some medications that relax the irritable bladder and some which reduce stress incontinence. Most medications come with a few side effects, but they give a lot of relief.

WHAT ABOUT SURGERY?

Almost all cases of SUI can be cured with surgery. There is, of course, medication you can take, but you can't take it before each time you cough or sneeze because you don't know when that's going to happen. And since there are simple and effective surgical treatments for SUI, we prefer to do that.

Of late, the way of treating SUI has changed a lot. Earlier, we used to just take care of it while doing surgery for prolapse. We would put stitches around the urinary outlet and tighten it and that would give the woman some degree of relief. But now we have some advanced treatments like:

Slings

A good surgery for stress urinary incontinence in females is a sling procedure. It consists of a synthetic mesh material in the shape of a narrow ribbon that is placed under the urethra through one vaginal incision and two small abdominal incisions. This adds strength to the weak pelvic floor muscles and provides support under the urethra.

The tension-free transvaginal tape (TVT)

This 20-minute procedure involves two tiny cuts and placement of a mesh tape underneath the urethra. It has a 80–95 percent cure rate.

The transobturator tape (TOT)

The transobturator tape (TOT) sling procedure provides support under the urethra. A mesh tape is fixed under the urethra through three small incisions in the groin area.

So every time the woman coughs, instead of the urine coming out, the outlet gets closed and she can't leak urine. This is a long-term solution. If a 20-minute procedure can rectify a problem that's so acute, the change in the woman's quality of life is pretty dramatic. Yet, women are not aware that there are solutions to such problems.

This is not the only way to treat the problem. There are over 50 surgeries to fix SUI. There is a laproscopic surgery where a camera is put inside the body and the joints between the bladder and the urethra are fixed with a tape. Unfortunately, I have observed that even doctors don't question their patients about SUI. They'll only deal with the problem that the patient comes with and won't check if there are other associated problems as well.

All doctors have had accidents of patients leaking urine all over us. We usually sit on a gynaecological examination table, at the foot end of the patient. As a typical test, we ask the patient to cough and almost every doctor has been caught unawares because the urine suddenly squirts out. But we've learnt our lesson now. We make it a point to always stand on the side and ask the patient to cough.

8

Endometriosis

ENDOMETRIOSIS IS A GYNECOLOGICAL CONDITION in which cells from the lining of the uterus (endometrium) start growing outside the uterine cavity, in the ovaries or around the uterus in the abdominal cavity. These endometrial cells are controlled by female hormones. In endometriosis, every time a woman has her period, there is bleeding inside the ovary or around the uterus in the pelvic cavity where these endometrial cells have abnormally placed themselves. The reason why endometriosis affects the ovaries is that they have the highest levels of hormones compared to any other organ in the body, and hence are the ideal environment for the growth of the endometrial tissue. Endometriosis is a condition that affects 10–15 percent of women during their reproductive years. Considering we have 12 periods in a year and if, for instance, the problem of endometriosis starts around the age of, say 28, the woman is going to suffer for many years as with each menstrual period, blood will accumulate in an area outside the uterus such as the ovary.

The disease progresses at a very fast pace and before you know it, large chocolate cysts are formed. They are called that because blood, after a period of time, starts to look like dark chocolate. Sometimes, we find large 8cm or 10cm cysts. And soon they'll start taking up the entire space of the ovaries. The ovaries are normally between 2cm to 3cm in size. And if inside a 2cm ovary there's a 10cm cyst, there's nothing left of that ovary. (See Fig. 9 in the insert pages.)

Several studies have shown that the incidence of endometriosis is much higher in women who have a sister or a mother suffering from the disease. A study carried out in Reykjavik by deCODE Genetics and Iceland's National University Hospital indicate that a woman is five times more likely to develop endometriosis if her sister has the condition, and even a cousin with the disease can raise the risk by more than 50 percent.

The causes of endometriosis are still unknown, although there are many theories. One theory suggests that during menstruation some of the tissue backs up through the fallopian tubes into the abdomen, a sort of reverse menstruation, where it attaches and grows. Other than genetics, women who'll give birth for the first time after 30 and women with an abnormal uterus are at the risk of developing endometriosis.

You are at a risk of developing endometriosis if:

- Your menstrual period started early.
- Your mother or sister has endometriosis.
- Your menstrual cycles are frequent and you bleed for a long time.
- You have never been pregnant.
- You have an abnormality from birth in the uterus that blocks menstrual flow.

Endometriosis is considered a non-cancerous cancer. The disease, of course, won't kill you, but it is very progressive and damaging. It's like an inflammation inside your body. In severe cases, which are becoming more common these days, all the organs in the pelvic cavity are stuck to each other. The tubes and the ovaries get stuck; then sometimes, the intestine gets stuck to that. There have been instances when we open up the woman to remove endometrial cysts and come across a jam inside the body. We just don't know where to begin. We call this situation a frozen pelvis. It means that everything is frozen and jammed inside. It's like a big ice block. We can't even put the laparoscope inside or differentiate where the uterus begins and the tubes end. That is, of course, an advanced stage of the disease. But we see a lot of damage even in patients who haven't reached that stage yet.

With every period cycle, there is an increase in the damage. For the woman, the menstrual period becomes very painful and the period pattern also changes. Because of the intense damage it causes, endometriosis can cause infertility. Endometriosis is one of the most common problems that gynaecologists currently face and it is responsible for a significant portion of gynaecological surgeries each year. It is one of the most complex and least understood diseases in our field and, despite many theories, we still do not have a clear understanding of its relationship to infertility.

What are the symptoms?

For many women suffering from endometriosis, severe pelvic pain is the main symptom. The pelvic pain typically starts to intensify before the period and increases in the next few days. After periods, the pain reduces. The amount of pain a woman experiences is not necessarily related to the severity of the disease—some women with severe endometriosis may experience no pain, while others with a milder form of the disease may have severe pain or other symptoms. Other symptoms of endometriosis include pain during passing stool or while urinating, premenstrual spotting, frequent or heavy periods, and pain during intercourse. Some women experience constant pelvic soreness or pain in the lower back that radiates down each leg. Other symptoms of endometriosis include:

- Spotting before the period.
- Irregular and heavy periods.

- Swelling and bloating in the lower abdomen.
- Blood in the stool during period.
- Infertility or difficulty in becoming pregnant.

Diagnosis

Endometriosis can be diagnosed clinically with sonography. You can see the endometriotic cyst on the scan and even the large size of the uterus can be picked up in a sonography. There's also a blood test tumour marker called CA125. It is usually used for ovarian cancers. But this is also elevated in endometriosis.

What's the solution?

Unfortunately, there is no permanent medical treatment for endometriosis. There is no way we can control this condition. Till the time the woman will have her period, she will continue to suffer. The only thing we can do from a medical standpoint is to stop the period. When a woman is younger, we can give her continuous contraceptive pills. Usually, a woman takes contraceptive pills for 21 days, then takes a break to have her period, and then continues them again. But in this case, she takes the pills for months and sometimes even years continuously without stopping to get her menstrual period. Continous use of progesterone hormone would also have the same effect. So when we stop the period, at least the disease won't progress. The disease is still there in the body, but won't cause the woman discomfort.

There is also a drug called GnRH Analog, which is one of the mainstays of the disease treatment. These are once-a-month or once-in-three-months injections which put the woman into menopause. They prevent the pituitary gland from secreting the controlling hormones FSH and LH. This stops the ovary from producing oestrogen. Once the body's hormones are down to the menopause level, there is no period. This gives the patient relief. But this also gives the woman all the symptoms of menopause like hot flashes and vaginal dryness. The moment we stop the drug and the period starts, everything goes back to the way it was. Typically, patients treated with GnRH Analogs will experience a relief in symptoms for a few years after which most patients experience a resurgence of symptoms. We bring about temporary menopause because we need to give the patients temporary relief. If I operate on a 28-year-old woman for the first time, by the time she is 32, she will again face the same symptoms and problems. And then I will again have to operate on her by the time she is 35. It's not wise to operate on a woman again and again. So I just try to delay the symptoms as much as possible with medicines.

All these surgeries are done laparoscopically and we are usually able to remove the disease, helping the patients do well for a couple of years. (See Fig. 10 in the insert pages.) Fertility is the main reason why this is done in younger patients. Fertility is always impaired in such patients. As soon as the surgery is done, we ask patients to immediately try to get pregnant—naturally or with IVF.

BUT HOW DOES ENDOMETRIOSIS AFFECT A WOMAN IN HER 40S?

We are talking about this disease in the 40s because it keeps coming back. So even though you may have had your first surgery in the 20s or 30s, we will eventually have to deal with them again in the 40s. If these women have been fortunate enough to see a pregnancy through this, they remain fine during that time because they don't have their menstrual periods during pregnancy. By the time the woman is done with the family, she's completely fed up because of multiple surgeries.

Along with endometriosis is a condition called adenomyosis. The only difference between this and endometriosis is that in adenomyosis there is bleeding within the walls of the uterus. So during every period, the bleeding takes place within the uterus. With every period, the uterus swells more and more and small pools of blood form within it. As the uterus becomes larger, it causes more and more pain to the woman because the uterus gets stretched every time she gets her period. I've known of women who are actually rolling on the ground because of the pain. Surgical treatment of adenomyosis is difficult as the disease is usually diffused. If the adenomyoma is localized in a part of the uterus, it can be removed surgically, though the surgery is complicated.

It's a disease that starts in the reproductive age group. A woman in her 40s has had adenomyosis for some years, fertility issues, and maybe even surgery for it. The uterus is probably large now and she's had pain for years. If the blood accumulation is localized, we can remove it by adenomyomectomy using a laparoscopic or open surgery. But in most cases the whole uterus is damaged. And the only treatment left is hysterectomy and to remove the ovaries as well. Usually, in a hysterectomy, we keep the ovaries in the body, but in this case there's no option but to remove them as ovaries are most often affected.

Endometriosis is most often found in the ovaries, but it can also be found in other places like the intestines, rectum, urinary bladder, vagina, cervix, vulva, and abdominal surgery scars. It's rare, but it happens. Almost 90 percent of endometriosis develops in the uterus. Since it's such a debilitating disease, this is the only condition where women look forward to menopause. Because once she has menopause, the disease will not progress and will slowly regress; the uterus will begin to shrink and she'll be a lot better off when she's fully into menopause.

9

Unplanned Pregnancies

UNPLANNED PREGNANCIES INCLUDE UNWANTED PREGNANCIES as well as those that are mistimed. Worldwide, according to the World Health Organisation, 38 percent of pregnancies are unintended.[1] That means about 80 million unintended pregnancies happen each year. Unplanned pregnancies result in about 42 million abortions per year, and 34 million unintended births.

While writing this book, I came across a story that may seem strange to you, but I, as a practicing gynaecologist, encounter such incidents almost every day. This couple from Britain had been trying for a child for over two decades. She was 26 when they started trying the natural way. But when nothing happened for many years, they tried IVF but that did not work either. By the time she was 42, they had given up their dream of starting a family. That's when the woman unexpectedly fell pregnant—not just once, but three times. At 47, she now has four children. In her interview, she talks about the shock and irony of it all. But I am not surprised. Women in their 40s have the second highest unplanned pregnancy rate after teenagers.

But how is that even possible? Many women believe that they can't get pregnant in midlife, or that the odds are slim. That is as far from the truth as possible. The fact is that fertility does start to decline each year starting from a woman's 30s. A healthy 30-year-old woman has about 20 percent chances of getting pregnant each month. By 40, the odds of becoming pregnant decrease to 5 percent each month. Despite these highly skewed odds, women can absolutely get pregnant in later reproductive years. We see cases of unplanned pregnancies in the 40s all the time.

Some scientists believe that this is because women of today's generation who are over 40 are more fertile than middle-aged women of previous generations—a change due to natural selection. They say that of the women who wait to try for a baby, only those genetically predisposed to longer-lasting fertility will be able to conceive. This gene is passed on to their children, who in turn can have babies later in life. Others also believe that some women have a brief burst of fertility as they approach menopause. It seems the body naturally stimulates the ovaries more aggressively as the number of eggs decline in an attempt to keep them working. This phenomenon, however, has neither been examined in great detail and nor has been confirmed.

What we do know for sure is that a woman is fertile

till she experiences menopause. Her fertility declines dramatically as her age progresses, but while there is always a chance that she can still have babies, a woman who is infertile has problems getting pregnant as she grows older. At the age of 45, a woman's periods are constantly irregular and they miss out on the pregnancy. A few days ago, a middle-aged Maharashtrian couple came to my clinic. The woman was 46-years-old. She said that she was getting irregular periods and thought that she was perimenopausal. She was having stomach pain, so she went for a sonography and found out that she was 24 weeks, i.e. 6 months, pregnant. The couple was left stunned because they hadn't expected it to happen; they already had a 20-year-old son. They came to me for an abortion. I told her I couldn't help her at all because 20 weeks is the legal cut-off for abortion in India. The couple too wasn't at fault because how could I have expected them to come to me sooner when they didn't even know about the pregnancy themselves? At 6 months, a woman's bump isn't that big. Most women pass it off as a bloated stomach from irregular periods. There's also a chance that since the woman hadn't had a baby in 20 years, she must've forgotten about the symptoms. She had no choice but to have the baby. I can understand why she didn't want the baby. Having a child in your 20s and 30s is very different from having a child in your 40s. There are things to consider like genetic disorders for the baby, higher risks for the mother, and how old the parents will be when the child is grown-up. They would also have to consider their long-term financial outlook. But I had no choice but to turn them away.

WHO'S TO BLAME?

One reason for the high rates of unintended pregnancy is women frequently stop using birth control in their 40s. Several studies have shown that roughly 25 percent women over 40 don't use contraception at all. A recent survey by the website 'Menopause Matters' revealed that 27 percent of premenopausal, 32 percent of perimenopausal, and 40 percent of postmenopausal women used no contraception at all. A lot of older women are probably too casual about contraception or not using it all, because they think that since they haven't been pregnant in over 10 years, there's no way it'll happen in their 40s. I have observed that women are scared of contraception and hence put the responsibility of it on to the husband. Unfortunately, there is not enough awareness about what contraception to use and for how long, especially when it comes to older women. And how do we reach out to a woman who is 40? Gynaecologists have no interaction with a 40-year-old woman. Women last meet a gynaecologist when they get pregnant. And once they have delivered their baby, they just disappear until some gynaecological problem comes up when they're older. Very few women come for annual check-ups in their 30s where we can advise and warn them about pregnancies in the 40s.

Contraception is extremely important in this age group because physically the woman finds it much harder to handle a pregnancy. In the 40s, a lot of women already have diabetes and high blood pressure. Pregnancy can aggravate that. And socially, in India, it is not really acceptable to have a child so late.

WHAT CONTRACEPTION OPTIONS ARE AVAILABLE?

Ross: We, we used a condom!
Rachel: I know, I know. But you know, condoms only work like 97 percent of the time.
Ross: Wha-what? WHAT? Well they should put that on the box!
Rachel: They do!
Ross: No they don't! (Storms off to his bedroom; pause; returns with a box of condoms in hand). WELL THEY SHOULD PUT IT IN HUGE BLOCK LETTERS!!![2]

Remember how Rachel gets pregnant in the hit sitcom *Friends* despite using contraception? The only way to prevent getting a blue line on the pregnancy test stick is to use the right contraception. But every contraception method can fail. Unplanned pregnancies can and will happen despite taking every possible precaution. Your husband may be using a condom and you may have a Copper-T inside your uterus—and you may still become pregnant. Gynaecologists have a cafeteria approach to contraception. We like to lay out a basket of options for women and see what works well for them. But the options are limited because, as I said before, there is no 'ideal' contraception. These are choices that have to be individualized to suit a woman's needs.

Most women choose from either the contraceptive pill, an intra-uterine device (IUD), or sterilization. Let's talk about the temporary methods first. Most women in India prefer temporary methods and, for some reason, permanent methods are on a decline in our country.

The pill

Contraceptive pills which are in a huge demand in younger women lose favour in women in their 40s. As women grow older, they become more concerned with the use of hormones. I have seen that women who had contraceptive pills when they were younger are scared to continue them in the 40s. Plus, a lot of women in the 40s may be diabetic or suffering from hypertension. Such women have to be very careful with their use of contraceptive pills. In diabetic women, hormone pills are known to change or worsen the control of diabetes. Women who have high deep vein thrombosis or suffer from migraines, liver disease, or gall stones are not ideally suited for contraceptive pills. When you're younger, you can get away with a lot of things. But when you are older, contraceptive pills have to be consumed under supervision.

The advantage of these pills is that they are extremely effective. If a woman is taking her pill properly and regularly, it is very unlikely that she will have an unplanned pregnancy. That cannot be said of most other contraceptive methods. Another advantage is that the woman is in control and doesn't have to include her partner in the decision making. Also, you can give them a break whenever you want to.

And, of course, the pill has many non-contraceptive benefits that are useful in the 40-plus age group. They regularize periods completely, which is very good because women in their 40s suffer from irregular periods. Lots of women also suffer from heavy bleeding and the pill works to stop that. If the bleeding is because of hormonal reasons, the pill will set it right. When you are on contraceptive pills, ovulation does not take place. So the period is also painless. Also, the pill ensures that your skin glows and reduces the ageing effect to some extent. It'll also help with adult acne.

There are many different varieties of the pill available these days. You can choose the combination depending on your requirement. There are low dose pills, ultra-low dose pills, and pills with only 20 micrograms of ethyl oestrogen, which makes them very, very low on hormones. These pills are to be taken for 24 days, instead of the usual 21-day cycle. Then, there are some pills that you have to take continuously for 3 months. That way, a woman will have her period only 4 times a year. This is very useful for women in India because most of us tend to suffer from anaemia. Not having her period for 3 months ensures that the woman doesn't lose blood every month and can stay strong and healthy.

Oestrogen patches

Another contraceptive option is the oestrogen patch. They used to be available in India a few years ago, but aren't right now. It's only a matter of time before they come back. They are to be worn like a band-aid on the lower part of the body and the hormones in the patch seep through the skin. The contraceptive patch works mainly by changing the body's hormonal balance so that the woman does not produce an egg every month. It also makes the cervical mucus thicker, which makes it difficult for sperm to get through to the uterus to fertilize the egg. The oestrogen patch also makes the lining of the uterus thinner, so it is less likely that a fertilized egg will be able to attach to the uterus. The patch has to be worn for 3 weeks. During the fourth week, when the woman is not wearing the patch, she should get her period. A lot of women are comfortable with oestrogen patches rather than taking a tablet every day.

Vaginal rings

Another option is the vaginal ring. It is a soft, flexible, plastic ring shaped like a bangle which contains hormones inside it. You have to insert the ring in the vagina on the third or fourth day of your period and it releases hormones. The vagina absorbs all drugs very well because it's a vascular area. The ring is kept inside for 3 weeks. It, thankfully, doesn't interfere with sexual intercourse and you don't have to remember to use it every day like you would with the pill. Most women don't feel the ring when it's inside. And it is, in a way, a lot safer than taking the oral pill. When you take a pill, it goes through your entire system, whereas if you take your hormones through the vagina or the skin patch, it doesn't go into your liver which can cause problems. The vaginal ring works better since it is closer to the uterus. There is also a much lesser quantity of hormones delivered into your body as compared to the pill.

IUDs and other devices

In rural India, a popular method of contraception is injectibles. These are progesterone-containing injections called Depo-provera to be used once in three months. Depending on your outlook, the positive or negative aspect of it is that the woman's periods will stop for three months. It's a very inexpensive injection, so women in rural India can afford it easily. The only negative aspect on these injectibles is that it takes about a couple of months for the period to come back to normal schedule.

Another option is the Copper-T, which is an intra-uterine device. There are two types of IUDs. One is Copper-T which is inserted into the uterine cavity and which acts as a physical barrier to pregnancy. The Copper-T is a T-shaped device with copper inside it. Copper prevents the embryo from implanting into the uterus because it has inflammatory qualities. Similarly, there's another IUD which is in the shape of a C that's mounted on a stick. It works the same way as a Copper-T. There's also a Copper-T that's coated with silver which lasts longer. These days, there are IUDs that can remain inside the uterus for up to 10 years.

It takes just two minutes to insert an IUD. But we always tell patients that after the first menstrual period, they should check if the device is in place. Sometimes, the uterus cramps and tends to push the device out. IUDs have a small thread that hangs out of the cervix. So the woman can check if the device is in place on her own and doesn't even need to visit the doctor for that. For women who need the period to feel normal, the IUD is perfect because they will continue to get periods. But a major disadvantage is bleeding disorders. Another side-effect is pelvic infection. That is why we never introduce a Copper-T in a woman who has never had a baby. It has to be noted that any IUD has a 4 percent failure rate. There are also more chances of an ectopic pregnancy occurring because since the IUD doesn't allow the pregnancy to settle into the uterus, it may move to the fallopian tube.

To counter the negatives of IUDs, hormone containing IUDs have been introduced. These are T-shaped devices with hormones present in the long arm of the T. Small quantities of progesterone is released very slowly into the woman's body over a period of five years. But it's slightly more painful to insert these devices into the body when compared to Copper-T which is why the patient may have to be sedated during insertion even though it take only a few minutes for insertion. In the first 2–3 months, the woman may encounter spotting on and off because the body is just getting adjusted to the hormone. But after 3 months, there is a continuous release of hormones and the lining of the uterus become very, very thin. It is not allowed to grow like it does for every menstrual cycle. As a result, the frequency of the menstrual cycle reduces over time and in many women, even stops completely. The advantage of hormone containing IUDs is that they give you long-term contraception and the failure rate is very less compared to a normal Copper-T. Also for older women, it has the advantage of reducing the heavy menstrual bleeding which is common in this age group.

Condoms

Apart from what I have mentioned above, there are also the mechanical methods of contraception. One of them is condoms. Condoms are the most commonly used contraceptive device in our country. That's because people are happy to use something that has no hormones, no side effects, and involves introducing no foreign substances in the body. Most people these days use medicated condoms. They have spermicide inside which kills the sperm present in the condom. Unfortunately, condoms are extremely ineffective if not used or removed properly. Sperms can leak out and condoms can rupture. If not stored properly, they may become weak and have perforations that can enable sperm to enter the vagina and cause pregnancy. That's why we recommend using another contraceptive method along with condoms.

There is also a female condom—an inverted condom—in which the V-shaped device goes into the vagina and the outer part covers the labia. Intercourse is done within the device, but most women are not comfortable doing that. Since it is cumbersome to use, it has somehow not taken off in a big way anywhere in the world.

These days the emergency pill has been gaining popularity. There are two types of emergency contraceptions available. What we used to do earlier is to give a high dosage of the normal contraceptive pill because it would change the environment of the uterus overnight and become unsuitable to handle a pregnancy. Now there is an individual tablet that contains a high dose of progesterone. When you take it within 72 hours of unprotected sex, the effect of the hormone on the lining makes it impossible to sustain a pregnancy. It makes the cervical mucus very thick and hopefully the pregnancy doesn't implant. The safety of the drug in terms of prevention of pregnancy is not that good. The sooner you take it after unprotected sex, the better it is. I wouldn't recommend older women to use this frequently because of the high amount of hormones it contains. Emergency contraceptive always disrupts the menstrual cycle. The woman may suffer from heavy bleeding. She won't know if she is pregnant because she's bleeding, making her think she's got her period whereas she could be pregnant with bleeding. If you have unprotected sex, another way out is to put in a Copper-T. It will work as an emergency contraceptive and then you shouldn't remove it and use it as normal contraception for the next couple of years.

STERILIZATION

If you aren't interested in taking your chances with an unplanned pregnancy, the foolproof way is to sterilize yourself. It is the only permanent way guaranteed to negate your changes of falling pregnant. Sterilization is typically done after a woman's period. That's because we want to completely ensure the woman is not pregnant. And it is only after her period that we'll know for sure she's not pregnant. If she comes to a doctor for sterilization in the 14th or 15th day of her cycle, she may have conceived and it's too early to show on a pregnancy test. There was a famous incident where a doctor had performed sterilization on a woman and subsequently she was found to be pregnant. She may have already been pregnant at that time, but it was too early and the doctor may have missed it. She went on to continue with her pregnancy. By the time she realized she was pregnant, she was already past the five month limit for abortion. She, of course, made quite a bit of noise about it, and there was a fair amount of media coverage on the incident.

But sometimes, a woman bleeds and she's not sure why that's happening. The bleeding could actually be pregnancy with bleeding which happens to so many women. Early in the pregnancy, some women bleed and believe that it's their period. So unless the doctor is 100 percent sure that the woman is not pregnant and performs a sterilization, the pregnancy may continue.

Also, sterilization can fail sometimes. It's been known to happen on several occasions. The failure rate is about 1 percent. That's why a patient always has to be informed that sterilization is not a guarantee against pregnancy. If you miss your period, always check for pregnancy. That's the primary reason we do sterilization post-period or soon after a delivery.

How does sterilization take place?

In women, the fallopian tubes are usually blocked in various ways to ensure that the egg cannot pass through, and hence the woman cannot become pregnant. The most popular method these days is laparoscopic tubal sterilization. You can either tie the tubes with a band or you can clip them with filshie clips, which are like tiny clothes peg clips. With filshie clips, the advantage is that you destroy a very small part of the tube, whereas the band destroys a large part of it. Some doctors even prefer to burn the tube with a bipolar current laparoscopically.

Before laparoscopy became very popular, all surgeries were done by an open operation. Sometimes, if a woman has already had 2–3 children, she wants to be sterilized as soon as she delivers so that there's no chance of another baby. Usually after delivery, the endometrium is very thick and the uterus is too large to introduce a laparoscope. So doctors make a tiny cut, less than an inch in size, just below the navel, and open out that small incision. Since the uterus is so large and elevated right after delivery, the fallopian tubes come easily into the picture. Doctors would then tie up the tubes with a thread and a needle. This method, though not used extensively in urban areas, is particularly popular in the rural areas because the latest technologies are often not available there. There's no guarantee you'll ever see that woman in your clinic again. So if she's come for her delivery and wants a sterilization, it makes sense to finish it all in one go.

For all sterilization procedures, we have to approach from the abdomen. We have to make a cut on the abdominal wall and that always has its risks. Since you are putting a sharp instrument into the body, it may injure the organs. So researchers were always looking for ways to do it naturally where you go through the vagina into the uterus, and try to block the tubes from inside. Many systems were devised, but none of the hysteroscopic procedures became popular, nor were they very effective either. Many years ago, doctors used to put quinine (a drug) into the uterus. It created a reaction that would block the tubes from inside. But the surgery wasn't very successful with that. Later on, doctors would also put in a plug on the tubes through the vagina. But there were instances of the plug coming off. The latest thing to come internationally—it still hasn't come to India though—is the Essure device. Here you approach the uterus from inside with a hysteroscope with a 1-inch spiral metal device. It is introduced through the uterine opening of the fallopian tubes. The device causes the tube to be inflamed and get blocked off. This is an expensive procedure but extremely safe.

What if you want to reverse the sterilization?

Even though sterilization is an irreversible process, sometimes patients do come in with requests to reverse the surgery. The process of reversing a sterilization is called recanalization. While recanalization success rates are not guaranteed, many surgeries are still successful. The success rate depends on how the sterilization took place. In sterilization with open surgery, a large part of the tube is removed. So if the woman wants a recanalization, the chances of success are very poor. In a laparoscopic sterilization surgery, the band destroys only a small part of the tube. And hence, it's easier to reverse it. But despite all the efforts, we may not succeed in opening up the tubes.

There are several reasons why a woman wants recanalization surgery. She may have lost a child and wants another one. Or she may have remarried and now wants a child with her second husband. It happens for religious reasons as well; Muslim women who have been sterilized cannot go on the Haj pilgrimage. I have had many patients come to me and want their tubes opened, not because they want a child, but because they want to go on the Haj pilgrimage. Recanalization is a much longer, harder procedure than sterilization. Closing the tubes is a 5 minute job. But opening the tubes is always a major procedure. The tubes are so fine and delicate that it takes a longer time to cut the part that has been damaged and resuture the tubes. And the opening is microscopic. We can't even see the canal of the tube with our bare eyes. Recanalization can either be done laparoscopically (which takes around 2 hours) or you can make a small bikini cut and cut off the part that has been damaged and align the tubes together. We use very fine prolene thread stitches. We can never give the patient the guarantee that the recanalization procedure will be successful. But it's safe to say that the woman has a 70 percent chance of conceiving naturally after the surgery.

The success of recanalization depends on several factors. One of them is the age of the woman. The body has seen much more wear and tear in an older woman. She may not be ovulating that regularly, or her husband's sperm count may have reduced. It also depends on the expertise of the surgeon. This is a specialized surgery; not every surgeon can do it very well. There are so many factors involved in having a child that the opening up of the tubes is just the first step. We first do an X-ray of the uterus to see till what level has the tube been blocked. If the tube is blocked very close to the uterus, chances of success are very less. If the tubes are blocked mid-way, the surgery usually goes very well. It's important to give it a lot of thought before you opt for sterilization.

What about sterilization in men?

Another option is vasectomy, the male version of sterilization. Vasectomy used to be very popular at one time in our country, but not anymore. It's a very simple and effective option. Unlike in women where you have to enter the abdominal cavity to sterilize her, vasectomy can happen even scalpel-free. During a vasectomy, the vas deferens (the main male duct through which semen is carried) from each testicle is clamped, cut, or sealed. This prevents the sperm from mixing with the semen that is ejaculated from the penis. An egg cannot be fertilized when there are no sperms in the semen. The testicles continue to produce sperm, but the sperm are reabsorbed by the body. An expert can do a vasectomy in 5 minutes and the process doesn't require hospitalization. But it's important to remember that the man doesn't become sterile immediately because there's already sperm stored in the system. After sterilization, multiple ejaculations have to take place. And only after the semen has been documented as not having any sperm is the man declared sterile. Vasectomy is very difficult to reverse. That's why we always ask a man to freeze his semen sample before going for a vasectomy if the couple wants a child later on. If the couple wants a child later and there's no semen sample stored, we can take the sperm from inside his body. His testes are still producing sperm; they just can't come out because the tubes have been blocked. We can remove the sperm from the testes with a fine needle and do a test tube baby procedure.

Termination

When all contraception fails, some women have no option but to go for a termination. While the methods of termination remain the same for all age groups, it is still important to know about it so that if you become pregnant unexpectedly in your 40s, you know what your options are.

For up till 7 weeks of pregnancy (which is counted from the first day of the last period), we are allowed to do a medical termination. We use a combination of drugs called RU486 or mifepristone and misoprostol over a period of 2 to 3 days. The first drug is an anti-hormone drug. It blocks the hormone and ensures that the pregnancy doesn't survive. It also blocks the hormone receptors and stops progesterone from reaching the uterus. The second drug contracts the uterus, which then pushes out the pregnancy. A combination of the two drugs works well. Either drug alone will not work. It works effectively in about 97 percent of women who will suffer from cramping and pain, bleeding, clots, and then have a miscarriage. There's no need to hospitalize a patient in such a case and the termination will happen at home. The actual abortion process takes about an hour.

The woman then continues to bleed for the next couple of days. Sometimes, bleeding may continue for up to two weeks, but it's very scanty. It takes that much time for the entire lining of the uterus to shed off. Since the uterus was getting ready for pregnancy, its lining is thicker.

This is what happened to a friend of mine. She is 40-years-old and called me five days before her vacation to Thailand. She told me that she had missed her period and a subsequent test showed that she was 6 weeks pregnant. She has children who are 8- and 10-years-old. She was not looking to have another baby, and was actually thinking more about the impending vacation. I immediately put her on the abortion pill. The pill worked really well for her and within 4–5 days when we did her ultrasound again, there was no trace of pregnancy.

But there are a few cases (3–5 percent) where the drug has either failed or there's a case of incomplete abortion. In such cases, there may be a blood clot or residue from the pregnancy still in the uterus. For that, we need to do a D&C or curetting. We open the cervix and put in a small device to scrape out the lining of the uterus. It's just like a manual evacuation.

If the woman is 12 weeks pregnant or under, we do a suction evacuation. We give the woman anaesthesia, and then dilate the cervix, which opens up into the uterus. We then insert the suction instrument and remove the pregnancy. This is a short process and takes about 10 minutes. If everything goes well, the patient can even go home in a couple of hours. Because this is a surgery, there is always a chance of complications. Since we use a sharp object, there is a possibility of an injury to the uterus. It can cause bleeding, or even a perforation in some cases. The object can go through the walls of the uterus and can injure the abdominal cavity and the intestines. There can even be an infection. This is more possible for women who've had a caesarean section. That's because once there is a scar on the uterus, it's more vulnerable to injuries.

In India, we are allowed to terminate a baby until 20 weeks of pregnancy. Between 12 weeks and 20 weeks, the pregnancy is much more advanced and it's difficult to remove it. From the second trimester, termination is just like a normal delivery. So if a woman is 4 months pregnant, we have to induce labour in her. There are different ways of doing it; there are labour inducing drugs and drips. There's even liquid medication that we can put inside the womb, which causes contraction and induces labour pain over 24 hours. This is a long process and requires hospitalization. The woman has to go through the trauma of delivering, and at the end not even have a baby to take home. The problem arises in a woman who's had, say, two C-sections in the past. For those patients to go through the labour process becomes risky because the uterus can rupture during the process. In those women, we have to do a mini C-section, also called a hysterotomy.

This is why no woman should take termination of pregnancy lightly. There's also a possibility of an ectopic pregnancy, where the pregnancy occurs in the fallopian tube. Here, there is no easy method of removing it. In all such cases, we have to do it surgically, either by putting in a laparoscope or via an open surgery. We either remove the pregnancy from the tube, or remove the tube itself. There is no easy treatment of ectopic pregnancy though in very early cases, we can give injections of a drug that can stop the ectopic pregnancy from growing. The injections may sometimes not work and eventually an operation maybe necessary.

A woman in her 40s has to go through the same procedures for termination as a younger woman. But the procedures are more risky at her age. I would strongly advise all women who are done with having children to use effective contraception because termination will not be a pleasant experience at all. Some women will also undergo a fair amount of psychological trauma because of termination of pregnancy. Some women are very matter-of-fact about the whole thing, but others are very emotionally traumatized. A lot of women take time to come to terms with this decision. That's why I recommend that they try really hard to not be in this situation.

10

Fertility

MOST PEOPLE FIND IT UNUSUAL talking about fertility when it comes to an older woman. That's because most people assume that by that age a woman is done having children. But the cross-section of patients that come to me—those who are pregnant or want to get pregnant—40 percent are over the age of 40. This is a huge number considering this is not a fertile period in a woman's life. But women are getting married late in life these days and are hence planning their children much later. They are deferring pregnancy in pursuit of a career. Of course, women are much more fussy now and just don't find the right partner. They won't compromise and will wait for the right person to come along. Sometimes, they find that person rather late in their life.

I have a friend who is 33-years-old. She got married a second time a year and a half ago. When she came to visit me, I thought she must be keen on having a baby. But she told me: 'I don't mind finding out if I am fertile, but I am not looking to have a baby right now. I have lots of things I want to do.' I was quite surprised and I advised her to prioritize this issue. I have met such women a number of times—women who've been married for about 5–7 years and are in their mid or late 30s, but are still not ready to have a baby. Ageing of the ovaries, however, does not wait and the eggs in the ovaries decline rapidly with age. Nowadays, since having more than one partner in a lifetime has become common in urban India, many women have had some sort of infection, sexually transmitted disease, or an abortion that may have caused pelvic infection and damaged their fertility. All these factors make it difficult for them to become pregnant when they are finally ready for it.

Smoking also affects your fertility. It is linked to 13 percent of infertility cases. Tobacco messes with your fertility in all kinds of ways—it makes your eggs deteriorate faster than they naturally would with age, increases your risk of early miscarriage and ectopic pregnancy, and can bring on early menopause (upto four years earlier, compared with non-smokers). Plus, if you end up needing in-vitro fertilization (IVF), smoking will reduce your chances of success by 34 percent. The encouraging news, though, is that once you do quit smoking, your fertility level will return to normal in about a year.

There are many other factors that affect fertility. Why has the woman not got pregnant till now? Are her tubes damaged? Is her uterus good or has it been exposed to infections? (See Fig. 11 in the insert pages.) All the problems that cause infertility in a younger woman cause infertility in an older woman as well. The woman could have damaged ovaries because of endometriosis, because of which she would've had a couple of surgeries. If she's had fibroids in the uterus or adenomyosis, the uterus would be damaged. If she's been exposed to chlamydial infections, her tubes may be blocked. Tuberculosis, especially in our country, may cause severe damage to the uterus, tubes, and ovaries. (See Fig. 12 in the insert pages.)

Similarly, in men, because of lifestyle changes like multiple partners, smoking, wearing tight clothes (which leads to decrease in sperm count), increase in temperature worldwide, working in warm environments, intake of drugs and certain strong medicines—fertility is adversely affected. These days cancer and cancer treatments are on the rise. Some younger men and women suffer from cancer which requires them to undergo chemotherapy and radiation. These treatments reduce the egg count in women and sperm count in men. Twenty years ago, there were hardly any cures for cancer. But with more treatment options these days, they survive and go on to have a normal life but the side-effect of cancer treatment is low fertility and so they have difficulty in conceiving. Another reason is that it takes a long time for patients to choose fertility treatment. They've been trying to get pregnant for some years. When nothing happens, they think of getting help. They go to their local doctor and try that treatment for a couple of years. By the time they come to an infertility specialist, they are that much older. Sometimes, women have had multiple miscarriages and it takes several months to get over a miscarriage and start trying again.

Every two years, after the age of 40, fertility is cut in half again. I don't want to sound alarmist, but I also don't want to make it sound like, 'Hey! You should count on being able to get pregnant', because you shouldn't count on being able to get pregnant. One of the major problems we encounter when a woman in her 40s wants to plan a baby is the ageing factor. At that age, the ovarian reserve is totally down and the egg quality and quantity have both reduced dramatically. Fertility starts to decline at the age of 27, and it goes down dramatically after the mid-30s. Most experts agree the fertility rate of women over 35 is about 10 percent each month, and at the age of 40 it drops to about 5 percent.

Sure, there are stories of actresses becoming pregnant late in life. One such example is Halle Berry. She fell pregnant at the age of 46 the natural way. But she's just been incredibly lucky. Not every woman will experience this kind of a miracle. I wouldn't want a 38-year-old woman to defer childbearing by taking such cases as a proof that she can easily conceive naturally in the years to come.

Natural pregnancies—when a woman is trying to get pregnant with her own egg—do occur in women in their mid-40s, but it would be nearly miraculous. Even in women using the assistance of IVF, there has never been a clearly documented case of a baby being born from an IVF pregnancy in a woman older than 45 years using her own eggs. The chances of having a baby at the age of 46 without intervention is probably about 0.01 percent or less. In such cases, there is no option but to seek fertility treatment.

So how do we go about finding a solution?

All women are born with a certain number of eggs, and you lose them over your reproductive life span. At some point—about 10 years before the onset of menopause—the number drops to a level where your fertility is compromised. So the first step in any assisted fertility treatment is to find out how many eggs a woman has. There are a couple of ways to do that. One of the commonest ways is to do a sonography. We will be able to count the exact number of antral follicles in the ovaries. These are the immature small size fluid circles seen in the ovary, which contain the egg. A follicle houses and nurtures an egg as it develops from an immature stage to maturity which occurs at ovulation, when the follicle bursts to release the egg. The more antral follicles you have, the more eggs you can produce. If you are considering an IVF treatment, the antral follicle count can give you and your doctor some idea about the number of eggs you can expect to yield.

The newer test to find out about the number of eggs is the Anti-Mullerian Hormone (AMH) test. It is a blood test which is a marker for the number of eggs in the ovaries. If the AMH is low, the woman's chances of getting a large number of eggs is less and hence the possibility of her becoming pregnant becomes much lesser. The older a woman gets, the more significance her ovarian reserve gets when it comes to fertility. If the AMH numbers are fine, the woman has a reasonably good chance of becoming pregnant with her own eggs.

Having said that, the quality of the woman's egg is also important. In the 40s even if she is producing eggs, they have a much lower chance of getting fertilized. And even if it does get fertilized, the chances of miscarriage are higher because the eggs are abnormal. At this stage, you can expect less fertility, a much higher rate of miscarriage, and a higher possibility of abnormal children, particularly with Down's syndrome.

What about the older husband?

Though men don't have a clearly defined stage like menopause in their lives, it has been proven that as they age, their fertility also reduces. There is DNA fragmentation inside the sperm, which is likely to result in the woman miscarrying their baby. Exposure to STDs may have caused their tubes, the vas, to be blocked. If the tubes are blocked, there will be zero sperm count because there is no space for them to come out. Also smoking, morbid obesity, medication, diabetes, and such other common problems can cause infertility in men.

Moving on

Once we have tested the woman's ovarian reserve and know that the woman can produce her own egg, we do routine investigations. We check her hormones and then test her for diabetes, cholesterol, high blood pressure, weight, etc. because older women face these problems. We then do a pap smear and mammogram, and eliminate the possibility of early cancer of cervix or breast before letting her into the fertility programme.

When she's been declared healthy, we put the woman on some drugs for ovulation because time is of essence here, especially if a woman comes to me in her late 30s or early 40s. I wouldn't want her to waste time in trying to get pregnant naturally. She may become pregnant naturally, of course, but we don't have the time to wait for that to happen, particularly for women who are marrying late. Usually, if the woman is younger, we let her try for one year before seeking fertility treatment. But for older couples, we give them about three months to try and get pregnant naturally. But if it doesn't happen, we put the woman on ovulation induction tablets. We try that for 2–3 cycles. If that is unsuccessful, there are injections to produce eggs because you have to give the ovaries a bit of a push. We give the woman tablets like Clomiphene and injections like Gonadotropins. From the ninth day of the period, we start monitoring the follicle to see if the egg is growing well. (See Fig. 13 in the insert pages.) When the egg is 18mm or

20mm in size, we inject HCG to rupture the egg. That's when we tell the couple to have planned relations so that the sperm can meet the ruptured egg.

The second method is intrauterine insemination (IUI). IUI is a simple and painless procedure wherein the husband's semen sample is taken and washed in the lab. The best quality sperms are picked up and inserted into the uterus of the woman. It doubles the pregnancy rate because the day the egg comes out of the ovary, it meets the sperm. This is one of the first things we do, provided the egg and sperm count are fine, the fallopian tubes are not damaged, and the uterus is ready to carry a pregnancy.

What if these treatments don't work?

As I mentioned before, we start with ovulation inductions, planned sexual relations, and IUI. None of these procedures should be done for more than 6 months in an older woman. But if she still doesn't conceive, we have to step up the treatment. If IUI doesn't succeed, we move on to In-vitro Fertilization (IVF) or the Intracytoplasmic Sperm Injection (ICSI) procedure. IVF is meant for women who have blocked fallopian tubes or unexplained fertility problems. ICSI is meant for husbands who have very low sperm count. The basic procedure for both treatments remains the same as far as the patient is concerned. It's just the lab technology that changes at the doctor's end.

For the woman, we first do a hysteroscopy to see if the

uterus is fine by inserting a small pencil like telescope with a camera inside her uterus through the vagina. This is a short and simple procedure. If there's a problem, we usually fix it in that same sitting. (See Fig. 14 in the insert pages.) Starting IVF, from the first or second day of her period, we start the woman on ovulation injections. (See Fig. 15 in the insert pages.) The idea is to produce a large number of eggs. The injections have to be taken for 10–12 days. In a younger woman, this procedure produces a large number of eggs. But in an older woman, it'll produce about 3–4 eggs. We monitor the growth of the egg through sonography. In about 11 days, the eggs are ready. By then, we give her the HCG injection to mature the eggs. A day later, we admit her to the hospital and suck out the eggs with a needle attached to the trans-vaginal sonography probe. The fluid which contains the microscopic eggs are sent to the laboratory and scanned for the eggs. The eggs, when seen, are isolated and kept in an incubator. Subsequently, the husband's semen sample is taken and the best quality sperms are dropped into the dish containing the eggs. The dish is left overnight just like that so the eggs meet the sperm. Fertilization can be seen in the culture dish. Two days later, depending on the growth of the embryo and its quality, 2 or 3 embryos are put into the womb of the woman. The woman is subsequently given hormone support to maintain the pregnancy. (See Fig. 16 in the insert pages.) Two weeks later, we conduct a pregnancy test. The woman doesn't need to take bed rest or stop working for this procedure to take place.

If the husband has a low or dismal sperm count, IVF will not work. For them, there's ICSI. In this treatment, the egg is retrieved from the woman the same way as IVF. (See Fig. 17 in the insert pages.) But the husband's sperms are individually picked up one by one by a hi-tech machine called the Micro Manipulator under high magnification. The machine has two needles. One needle holds the egg and the other needle picks up the sperm and injects it into the egg. The procedure that follows is the same as IVF.

A treatment that's more advanced than ICSI is Intracytoplasmic Morphologically-selected Sperm Injection (IMSI). It can be taken by men who have very low sperm count or in those cases where the woman has had recurring miscarriages because of abnormal sperms in the semen. Using ICSI, the sperm you see under a regular microscope is just a tiny little dot moving around. This only helps you distinguish a live sperm from a dead one. But with IMSI, we have the ability to magnify the sperm 7,000 times and you can even distinguish a normal sperm from an unhealthy one.

A lot of men get very shocked when they hear that they have zero sperm count, which is also known as azospermia as otherwise they may be perfectly normal and healthy. A common reason for zero sperm count is congenital absence of the vas which is a birth defect. In such cases, the testes produce sperm, but the tubes that transport the sperm are absent. We do a blood test for FSH to find out if the testes are normal and not in failure. If the FSH is normal, we can retrieve the sperm from the the testes directly with a testicular biopsy. With the help of needles, a small amount of tissue is removed from the testes which contains the sperm. These sperms are used by ICSI or IMSI to fertilize the egg. There was an Italian study in 2008 involving 446 couples in which the male was infertile but the woman had no perceivable fertility problems. The pregnancy rate among the IMSI couples was 32.9 percent as opposed to 26.5 percent among the couples who used ICSI.[1] With these two technologies, many men with zero sperm count have been able to have children of their own. Of course, if there is total testicular failure and no sperms are found even on biopsy, then the couple has to resort to using donor sperm or then opt for adoption.

Despite all this cutting-edge technology at our disposal, the success rate of IVF in an older woman is still less when compared to a younger woman. In a woman in her 40s, the covering of the embryo is also very hard and thick. That's why it sometimes doesn't rupture and the pregnancy doesn't implant. For these women, it sometimes helps to do laser hatching. The embryo's outer layer is cut before you put it inside the womb, using a laser. It's much finer than the laser used on the eye.

Another technique that's gaining popularity is blastocyst culture. A blastocyst is a five-day-old embryo. Normally, we put the embryo into the woman's uterus by day 2 or 3. But it has been found that if you keep the embryo in the culture for 5 days, it is much more mature and it increases a woman's chances of pregnancy.

WHAT IS THIRD PARTY REPRODUCTION?

Sometimes, when you and your husband can't make a baby on your own, a third party is involved in the making of a family. There are various permutations and combinations that take place for us to arrive at third party reproduction as a solution. If the husband has normal sperm count, but the woman is not able to develop eggs, the only way to get her pregnant is by borrowing eggs from another woman. Egg donation gives excellent outcomes because the only problem here is the absence of egg. And when you take a young woman's egg, you bypass that problem. In our country, it is legal to use an anonymous egg donor with the condition that the donor has to be married and have children. The donor also has to undergo all the necessary health check-ups and if everything is normal, she's introduced into the egg donation programme. The donor will have to go through the entire IVF procedure. Once the donor's eggs are given to the doctor, they are inseminated with the husband's sperm. At this time, the recipient woman's uterus has to be ready to start her pregnancy. We suppress her hormones completely with an injection. And then we give her hormone tablets to build up the lining of the uterus, so it's ready to carry a baby. Once that's ready, we give the woman progesterone and the embryo is implanted into her womb.

Recently, I had met a couple where the woman's AMH was less than 0.1 and the husband had practically no sperm. I had to tell them that their chances of becoming pregnant even with IVF were dismal but they still wanted to try. We gave her very high drugs to stimulate her ovaries to produce eggs, but they didn't work. So we opted for embryo donation. In certain situations, where there are problems with the husband's sperm as well as the woman's eggs, we opt for embryo adoption or embryo donation. The egg and sperm are both from donors and an embryo is created in the lab and that is implanted in the womb of the woman.

These techniques are used in older couples. This is also how a menopausal woman conceives. There are so many incidents that we read in the newspapers about 50- and 60-year-old women having a baby. In such cases, a woman's periods are restarted. We give the woman hormone pills for 21 days and then stop them. This cycle is continued for about 3 months and her periods starts again. This way, the uterus that had shrunk due to the onset of menopause will start to grow in size and get ready to carry a pregnancy. After her period has become regular, we do a hysteroscopy and check if the uterus is fine. We also do a thorough medical examination of the woman, including a psychiatric evaluation to see if the woman is mentally capable of having a pregnancy. And then, we take a readymade embryo and put it inside her womb. By egg donation or embryo donation, the woman can get pregnant.

WHY WOULD AN OLDER WOMAN WANT A CHILD?

There are many women who ask me why an older woman, say in her 50s, needs to have a child at her age. But what they don't understand is that no woman is going to have a child at 50 just for fun.

I have so many stories where women are so desperate to have a child. About two years ago, I had six people come into my clinic. They were the relatives of a 50-year-old woman and her 60-year-old husband. The woman had just lost her 20-year-old son, her only child, in a motorbike accident. She was begging me to give her another child and her husband was literally touching my feet and requesting me to help them. The woman was extremely depressed because of the death of her son and had even attempted suicide. We did IVF on her and she went on to have a healthy baby and it was an amazing experience even for us. They came to visit me a year after the baby's birth and were so happy. The woman was now busy raising their daughter and the couple had something to live for. Such women do very well with the whole procedure because they are so desperate to have a child.

Surrogacy is another option which can be used in unique cases where a hysterectomy has been done or the woman is born without a uterus. Also, if the woman is unable to carry a child due to health reasons or has had many miscarriages, surrogacy provides a solution. The surrogate contributes nothing except the right environment for the baby to grow in.

There's another couple my husband and I know whose 16-year-old daughter died of pancreatitis. To say that they were devastated by her death would be an understatement. The mother was 44 at that time and had already been menopausal for 4 years. The woman used to live in the suburbs of Mumbai and the husband in south Mumbai because he worked there. They used to meet only on weekends and wanted another child desperately. But she was menopausal and had a large sub-mucous fibroid. It hadn't bothered her so far because she was in menopause. But now that she wanted a baby, it would be a hindrance. I started her on hormone pills and she got her periods back. I then shaved off her fibroid using operative hysteroscopy surgery. We borrowed an egg from a donor and used her husband's sperm and did IVF. She got pregnant in the first cycle and delivered a baby girl. Since she'd lost a daughter, she kept saying that her daughter had come back. The child is 2-years-old now. My husband and I were invited to her first birthday party. I couldn't go, but my husband attended. We usually don't attend such functions, but these patients were special. Their entire chawl had been lit up and as soon as my husband reached, they burst firecrackers. They called him up on a pandal and everyone clapped for him. It was such an emotional moment that even though he has helped thousands of couples have babies, he was in tears. There are so many stories like this which keep us going. The case had really moved us emotionally, and we didn't charge the couple any money for the procedure.

While there is no law in India on ART, there are guidelines we have to operate by. A lot of expert inputs have gone into the making of the guidelines. And those guidelines do allow for surrogacy and egg and embryo donation in India.

Why you shouldn't delay IVF?

There's a reason why I stress that we shouldn't lose any time in starting fertility treatment in an older woman. A patient just came to me , again in her 40s, as she had blocked tubes. She had done her recanalization process twice to try to open her tubes. That's never recommended. But she must've been really keen to have children and wanted to take her chances. But her tubes didn't open and she has still not conceived. So instead of wasting precious time, the best thing for her to do is IVF. She should've gone for that immediately after the first recanalization surgery failed.

A few weeks ago, a 40-year-old woman came to my clinic. She had been married for 5 years and had been trying to get pregnant for the last 3 years. She first conceived and had a miscarriage at 5 months. Then she fell pregnant and miscarried again at 3 months. The third time she lost the baby at 5 weeks. She had been seeing another doctor all this while and was sent to me on recommendation. I was very surprised to see that even though she was 40, no other doctor had told her to do a laparascopy and hysteroscopy. An X-ray showed that she had a bicornuate uterus, which means she had 2 small uterei instead of one normal sized one, and this was a birth defect. One of her fallopian tubes was completely blocked, probably because of the miscarriages. Despite all these problems and her age, she was just having one simple tablet to increase ovulation and had been trying to conceive naturally. She was going about it the wrong way. Her AMH value was 0.3, which is absolutely pathetic. This means she was not producing any eggs, except for one odd egg here and there. I told her that her time was running out and within a year she would have no eggs left. And even if by some miracle she does get pregnant, she wouldn't be able carry it to term because her small uterei means they won't be able to hold the pregnancy. I told her that there's a possibility she has a septum or a curtain in the uterus and not 2 separate uteri. A septum can be removed by a half-hour surgery and the problem of recurrent miscarriages can be solved. And if tests confirm that there's no septum and she just has two uterei, we can consider surrogacy. She has to do something radical if she wants a child. And surrogacy is a great option. It's better than trying for a year more, by which time she may not even produce a single egg. But even at this stage, despite so many disappointments, it's hard for her accept that this is what she needs to do. Women sometimes are so resistant to solutions that are suitable for them, they fail to see time is running out.

11

Gynaecological Cancers

Cervical cancer

Did you know that more women in India die from cervical cancer than in any other country? Cervical cancer kills around 72,000 women in India every year, more than 26 percent of the 2.75 lakh deaths worldwide. The 40s is the most important age for cancers in women and that is when we start investigating for cancer. Cancer, of course, can happen to anyone. But gynaecological cancers are rare in women who are in their 20s and 30s. The moment a woman turns 40, we ask her to do the basic screening for cancer.

For a long time, doctors didn't know why a woman would be afflicted with cervical cancer. But now we know that a majority of the cases are caused by the human papilloma virus (HPV) and is related to poor genital hygiene and infections. There are over 200 types of HPV, but only a few strains cause cervical cancer. If a woman has strain 16 or 18 of HPV, the chances of her getting cervical cancer is extremely high.

Who can suffer from cervical cancer?

In other cancers, it's difficult to point out the causes. But we have the answers with cervical cancer. It is often not genetic though it may be seen in families, maybe due to similar lifestyles. Women who marry early, have many children, or have multiple sexual partners are more likely to get cervical cancer. Women with lower immunity due to diseases like HIV are at a very high risk for cancer of the cervix. Women on long term contraceptive pills and smokers may also be at a higher risk. Cervical cancer is a very slow-growing cancer. The exposure to cancer may begin in the 20s, but the disease may not be diagnosed till late 30s or 40s. We've had several 25-year-olds who are surprised when we ask them to do a pap smear for cervical cancer. But they may be unaware that the disease may have already started growing in them. So a pap smear will let us know if she has very early cancer and we can pick up a high-risk group much earlier.

HPV testing is fairly new in India; it came here only about 2 years ago. But before that, a pap smear was still useful because we could still pick up some abnormality in the cells that could one day lead to cervical cancer. Since it's usually a slow growing cancer, we could still pick up cervical intraepithelial neoplasia (CIN), which is a very early and localized stage of cervical cancer. The cervix is a tube and the cancer usually starts from the inside of the tube. Young girls usually have CIN Stage 1 or 2.

The symptoms of cervical cancer are vaginal discharge, foul smell, intermenstrual bleeding, and bleeding after intercourse. However, in early stages there are no symptoms.

The cervical cancer jab

Now we know why cervical cancer happens and that there are good tests to detect it, making it an easily preventable cancer. There is no treatment for HPV, but there are drugs that prevent it from becoming active. We also have the cervical cancer vaccine. Ideally, the vaccine should be given at a young age. So if a woman is vaccinated before she is sexually active, then you're really protecting her. It's usually given at the age of 12. But the company that manufactures the vaccine says that it can be given even up to the age of 42 for some degree of protection.

How do we screen the woman?

When a woman comes to us at 40, we first suggest a pap smear. We don't always test for HPV because it's expensive and not every woman is at a high risk of HPV. If the woman has a history of multiple sexual partners, we definitely suggest testing for HPV. We also examine the cervix by exposing it using an instrument, and visually check if the cervix has been eroded. In such cases, the skin comes out and the area looks red. Sometimes, we can see small cysts and ulcers on the cervix. Sometimes, there is even a small growth in the shape of a cauliflower on the cervix, meaning something's wrong. Then we do a pap smear. With the help of some cotton swab or a small brush, we enter the cervical canal and scrape the lining of the cervix. We put that sample on to a slide and send it to the lab for analysis. The test results will show us if there are any abnormalities in the sample that may be a sign of a disease. At the same time, we can also test the patient for HPV. It is done just like the pap smear with a brush being inserted into the cervical canal. And since this is a live culture that we extract, the lab tests it differently.

If the pap smear shows some abnormalities or the cervix looks unhealthy during the physical examination, we do a slightly more detailed test called the colposcopy. It is done with the help of a telescope that has a camera attached to it. It magnifies the area inside the cervix. With this, we can apply certain solutions like iodine on the walls of the cervix, and depending on the colouration the cervix takes on, we know if it is an infected or abnormal area. The camera and magnification enable us to see the blood vessels of the cervix properly. And if the blood vessels show a particular pattern, we know that the woman is at risk for cervical cancer. A certain expertize is required to do a colposcopy; it's not a test every doctor can do. A colposcopy also gives us more information on where to take a biopsy from. If you look at the cervix head-on, it looks like a ring that is one-inch wide. And the entire area may not be cancerous. With a colposcopy, you can zone into one area that looks infected and can take a tiny biopsy from there for testing. A biopsy is the final test for diagnosis of cervical cancer. We can also do a four-quadrant biopsy, wherein we take a tiny piece from all four corners of the cervix and send those samples for analysis. Sometimes, we also scrape out a bit of the endometrium of the uterus while we're checking out the cervix to know if the cancer has spread there too.

How is it treated?

Once the woman has been diagnosed with cervical cancer, the treatment will depend on how far the cancer has spread as well as the type. Most cancers of the cervix are squamous cell type but some maybe adenocarcinomas. The ability to spread rapidly depends on the type and grade of cancer. In all cancers, the stage where it's at is very important. Stages like 1, 1a, 1b, 2, 2a, and 2b are allotted, so that all doctors are on the same page as far as the diagnosis and hence the treatment is concerned. If the patient is at the CIN stage, then we can do a conisation where you drill out the entire core of the cervix, remove the parts that are affected, and not touch the other areas. Here, the cervix will be damaged to some extent because we are removing a part of it. Even for cervical cancer that's detected, in early stages, we have to do a radical surger, where the uterus and the areas surrounding it are removed. That is called Wertheims hysterectomy. The patient may require radiation therapy if the cancer has spread further. If the cancer has spread and moved into the neighbouring areas, it becomes inoperable. Then, we can't do any surgery and radiation and chemotherapy are the only treatment. But those come with their own side-effects. This is why it's important for the cancer to be detected early. When we tell women to get screened, they aren't receptive to the idea and insist that they are healthy and fine. They blame doctors saying that we are only interested in making money. But the reason we ask for those tests is because we want to pick up something early that may become deadly someday.

In India, there's still a lack of awareness about cervical cancer and hence not many women will get themselves screened. That's why so many women suffer from it. If I am not mistaken, 1 woman dies of cervical cancer every 7 seconds.

Uterine cancer

We now move up the body from the cervix to the uterus. A lot of women are unaware that there's something called the cervix in their body and that it's different from the uterus. Uterine cancer is completely different from cervical cancer. Nineteen out of 20 uterine cancers are cancers of the endometrium, the inner lining of the uterus. This is called endometrial cancer. It is the most common type of uterine cancer. The remaining 5 percent are tumours of the outer muscular lining called sarcomas.

The typical woman who acquires endometrial cancer is a 'fat, female at 40'. She's overweight, very often diabetic, and may not have had children or maybe infertile and probably started periods early and may achieve late menopause. Endometrial cancer is caused by hormonal issues. Any woman who is exposed to uncontrolled oestrogen in the uterus has a higher risk of suffering from this cancer. So a young girl with PCOS, if she is not careful and has irregular periods for many years, can go on to have endometrial cancer when she's in her 40s. Most endometrial cancers appear after menopause, and the risk continues to climb with each successive decade. About 95 percent of these cancers occur in women over the age of 40.

Why fat, 40, female?

The problems of PCOS are the classic problems of endometrial cancer as well. Women who suffer from irregular and delayed periods have an endometrium that's continuously growing (normally, it sheds every month). PCOS patients usually get very late periods. Also, patients who have chronic anovulation are likely to suffer from uterine cancer. In a normal menstrual cycle, oestrogen is released in the first half of the period, after which ovulation takes place and progesterone is formed. Progesterone is a balancing hormone and prevents the growth of the endometrium. In anovulatory patients, the oestrogen keeps coming out and ovulation doesn't take place, so the egg doesn't come out of the ovaries. So the entire time, only oestrogen is acting on the uterus and the stabilizing effect of progesterone hormone doesn't come in at all. This keeps happening for a long period of time and the endometrium keeps growing. Similarly, women who are extremely overweight produce a lot of oestrogen in their fat as not only are the ovaries producing oestrogen, even the fat is producing oestrogen. Overweight women are 3 to 10 times more likely than average to develop endometrial cancer, depending on how much extra weight they are carrying and how long they have carried it. When a woman is 40 and a sonography shows that her endometrium is very thick, we have to investigate it immediately. For menopausal women, the endometrium should not be more than 2mm–4mm thick. If it's thicker, we have to check for cancer.

What's the best way to fight it?

It is, however, important to note that every thick endometrium is not cancerous. That condition is called hyperplasia when the endometrium becomes too thick. It is not cancer, but in some cases, it can lead to cancer of the uterus. The best precaution against uterine cancer is an annual pelvic sonography. That's the only way to know if a woman who doesn't have obvious symptoms is suffering from endometrial cancer.

If the sonography shows the presence of something abnormal, we have to start with the diagnosis. Back in the days, we used to do only a dilatation and curettage (D&C). We'd put an instrument into the uterus, scrape out the lining, and send it for a pathological diagnosis. But now, rather than do a blind D&C, we prefer to look inside the uterus with a telescope and camera that's attached to it. That way, we can even encounter growths like polyps or fibroids in localized areas. (See Fig. 18 in the insert pages.) Once we find out what the unhealthy areas are, we take a biopsy. What we're ideally looking for is a test result that says simple hyperplasia. It's a swelling that's not cancerous and can be reversed through medication. The woman can take 12 days of progesterone tablets every month for a few years or can have a progesterone containing intrauterine device inserted which delivers progesterone hormone into the uterus for 5 years. These can control the hyperplasia and prevent it from progressing. Some patients have complex hyperplasia, which is a pre-cancerous stage. We can treat that either with hormonal therapy or remove the uterus as a preventive condition. But if you miss these stages and directly pick up endometrial cancer, we have to find out what stage it is at. Depending on the stage and type of cancer, we can start treating it. The typical treatment is a hysterectomy with removal of the ovaries. These days, women are going in for radical surgeries where lymph nodes and any other tissue affected by cancer is also removed. Sometimes this is followed by hormonal therapy or chemotherapy.

Ovarian cancer

Ovarian cancer is the most dangerous and the most difficult to diagnose. A woman of any age group can have ovarian cancer, though it usually occurs in women who are older than 50. But they have been known to happen to women in their late 40s as well. The ovaries are very small—typically about 1 inch in size—and are located deep inside the pelvis. A woman suffering from uterine or cervical cancer will always bleed through the vagina. That's how we know something's wrong. Ovarian cancer is often termed a silent killer because its symptoms do not cause alarm amongst women until it has reached an advanced stage. The only symptom a woman may have is gas and indigestion, unless the cancer is at a very advanced stage. Since the ovaries are so small, they will grow to a fairly large size before they are picked up. (See Fig. 19 in the insert pages.) Doctors will also realize there's a problem only when the abdomen is bloated and you can see the stomach bloated because the tumour has grown big and there is fluid accumulation in the area. Almost all cases of ovarian cancer are picked up in the advanced stages.

An article in *USA TODAY* says that researchers in the US who are trying to develop a diagnostic tool for ovarian cancer are hoping that dogs' keen sense of smell will help. The article titled 'Dogs trained to help sniff out ovarian cancers' says, 'An early detection device that combines old-fashioned olfactory skills, chemical analysis, and modern technology could lead to better survival rates for the disease, which is particularly deadly because it's often not caught until an advanced stage. Using blood and tissue samples donated by patients, the University of Pennsylvania's Working Dog Center has started training three dogs to sniff out the signature compound that indicates the presence of ovarian cancer.'[1]

Who are at risk?

The cause of ovarian cancer is not known. Older women who have not had children, and those who have close relatives with ovarian cancer are at an increased risk. Some women who have a strong family history of breast and ovarian cancer may carry the BRCA1 and BRCA2 gene which puts them at very high risk of developing these cancers. Women who have used contraceptive pills for a long time have a much reduced risk of developing ovarian cancer.

How is it diagnosed then?

The diagnosis of ovarian cancer is done by sonography. You can also do a colour Doppler at that time. It is a procedure used to examine the blood vessels and shows how much blood is going to the ovaries. If something is amiss, it will show up. Once you think that there is a high suspicion of ovarian cancer, an MRI is the best way to go. It is a very accurate test and will tell us if there is an ovarian tumour and also if the cancer has spread. It will pick up lymph nodes and affected tissues in the other areas as well. These tests will tell us about the presence of fluid. Fluid is always a bad sign because it means that the cancer has spread in the abdominal cavity. Fluid collection is called ascites. We can also aspirate the fluid with a needle under ultrasound control and check the fluid to see if it contains cancer cells.

Once we feel that there could be a possibility of a tumour, or even better as a screening test, we use ovarian tumour markers. These are blood tests. One of the commonest ones is CA125. Other tests are CEA, Alpha Feto Protein, and HCG. These days there's a new tumour marker called HE4. This gives more accurate results.

How do we treat ovarian cancer?

The treatment of ovarian cancer is usually debulking where we remove as much of the tumour as possible. The uterus, tubes, ovaries, omentum, etc are all removed during surgery. Ovarian cancer often responds very well to chemotherapy. Whether it's done before or after surgery depends on individual cases. During the surgery, we can also do a frozen section. While we operate to remove the cancer, we remove a piece of the tissue or the entire ovary and send it to the lab for an urgent diagnosis. A pathology report takes 5 days, so we don't know how much of the area to operate. Frozen section is an instant pathology report and within 20 minutes one can know if a woman is suffering from cancer, and you can proceed with the surgery accordingly.

Breast cancer

Breast cancer is the most common cancer worldwide. In India, however, cases of cervical cancer are still more than breast cancer. I don't know if incidents have been increasing or that we're diagnosing them early, but breast cancer cases are on the rise everywhere. It tends to occur at an earlier age than other cancers or heart attacks. Chances of developing breast cancer rise dramatically as women age—up to age 39, the chances of getting the disease are about 1 in 231; from age 40 to 59, the risk has gone up to 1 in 25.

There are certain kinds of breast cancers that are hereditary, like Angelina Jolie's cancer scare because of the presence of the BRCA gene that runs in her family. Women with the BRCA gene usually suffer from both breast and ovarian cancer. Earlier this year, Angelina Jolie began a global discussion on preventative therapies towards breast and ovarian cancer with the revelation that she underwent a double mastectomy. Following the death of her mother at 56 to breast cancer, Angelina chose to have the genetic test to see if she had any BRCA mutations. With that history in mind and finding she did have BRCA mutations, her risk is above average. Predicted to have about an 87 percent chance of getting breast cancer and a 60 percent chance of getting ovarian cancer, Angelina opted to remove both her breasts as a first step towards reducing her risk of breast cancer alone. She now has a less than 5 percent chance of developing breast cancer. Removing her ovaries is perhaps a more complex decision, a decision that requires a fine balance of timing. Removing the ovaries in a pre-menopausal woman, a surgery known as an oophorectomy, will push the woman into early menopause, which comes with several adverse side-effects such as osteoporosis and a general decline in well-being. This decision can have a profound effect on the health of the woman. And that is not even the full extent of BRCA mutations and cancer. This traumatic surgery will not reduce the risk of peritoneal, pancreatic cancer or melanoma; all are cancers that can develop with alterations found in these two genes. But this is particular only to this mutation of gene.

Why cancer isn't always inherited?

A lot of women don't test themselves for cancer because no one in their family has it. But cancer has to start somewhere and you could be the first person that gets it in your family. That's why we recommend that every woman after the age of 40 starts breast self-examination after her menstrual cycle. Post period, the breast is soft; it's not heavy or tender like it was before your period. You have to check both your breasts, the armpits, and check if there's any discharge from the nipples. You also have to see if the texture of the skin on your breasts has changed.

The only problem with breast self-examination is that only a big lump can be felt with the hand. Any lump that's smaller than 2cm will go undetected and by the time you go to the doctor, it's already too late. That's why while breast self-examination is good, it's not the answer to detection of cancer. I think it's a better idea to start doing mammograms. There is a debate in the US about what is the right age to start. While most women start going for mammograms from their 40s, some doctors say that that's too early and after you hit 50 is the right time.

Why are mammograms important?

Breast cancer can be extremely malignant. That's why annual checks should be conducted. Along with a mammogram, you should do a sonography as well because a sonography will pick up certain irregularities that a mammography doesn't. Most women are scared of a mammography because they think it's painful. Yes, it is painful because the breast is squeezed between two X-ray plates. But that pressure lasts for barely half a minute. If for those 30 seconds of pain, you can avoid a lifetime of the pain of cancer, I don't see any problem in it. It would help if you do the test after your period because it'll hurt a lot less.

In a pre-menopausal woman, a lot of times the result of a mammogram will say that she has dense breasts. Dense breasts are more prone to cancer because you can't see through them properly and hence may miss a small cyst or lump. You may miss a microscopic lump called a microcalcification. The lump is called that because it is a small deposit of calcium. A mammograph will pick up a particular kind of microcalcification.

The next stop is a biopsy to check if a cyst or tumour is cancerous. Using a needle, fluid is removed from a cyst to check if it contains cancerous cells. This requires either a needle biopsy, a core biopsy, or a surgical biopsy to be performed. For a needle biopsy, a fine needle is inserted into the lump and cells are drawn out. In a core biopsy, a sample of breast cells and tissues is removed for examination. A surgical biopsy is an operation that removes the whole lump and some normal tissue around it. Tru-cut biops is available in India now. A thick needle is inserted into the suspicious area of the breast and it has a device that cuts off the tissue. So you aren't sucking out a few cells like other biopsies, but cutting out an actual piece of the tissue.

When's a mastectomy required?

In early stages of breast cancer, just the tumour or lump can be removed (lumpectomy). In patients with a tumor smaller than 4cm, lumpectomy may be an effective treatment or removal of larger amounts of breast tissue may be necessary. Removal of the entire breast is called mastectomy.

If the tumour is detected very late, we may have to do a mastectomy and remove the entire breast and the armpit tissues. This is a very dramatic surgery, not just for cosmetic reasons, but also because during the operation, the lymph nodes in the axilla are removed. This has the side-effect of causing lymphedema (swelling) of the arm on the same side, as the removal of lymph nodes reduces lymphatic fluid drainage. Breast implants after the mastectomy are usually done at the same surgery. Radiation therapy may be required in some women with breast cancer. Patients with estrogen receptor positive tumors are given long-term hormonal therapy. The patient is often put on a drug called Tamoxifen to prevent recurrence of the cancer. But in a woman who has a uterus, it can cause endometrial hyperplasia. Very often, a woman with breast cancer is put on Tamoxifen and she gets post-menopausal bleeding and thickening of the endometrium. In such a case, we have to check the endometrium to see that there's no development of cancer. I had a patient about a year ago who was 26-years-old and about to get married. She incidently found a lump in her breast one day which turned out to be cancer. She had come to me because she wanted to preserve her eggs. That way she could pursue chemotherapy and radiation without worrying about whether she'll have children someday. A lot of women are going for such options. You can even freeze your entire ovary. All your decisions depend on your level of awareness. If you have all the information, you'll ensure you follow that path that gives you more options for the future.

ANNUAL SCREENING AT 40 FOR CANCER

Every woman after turning 40 should go for these tests annually.

- Pap smear.
- Trans-vaginal sonography. It looks at your cervix and uterus and checks for fibroids and tumours, if there are any.
- CA125 blood test.
- Mammography.
- Bone density. If we see that the bones are weak, the patient can start preventive therapy. It's difficult to reverse weak bones, but we can definitely prevent them from becoming weaker.

12

Non-gynaecological Issues

I'VE NOTICED THAT AS PEOPLE get older, they become more stubborn and are unwilling to change the way they've been living for so many years even when it's risky to not do otherwise. They'd rather take their chances with the disease than doing their best to prevent it. But you have to find a way to make sure you're healthy every day and seek help when there's one of these problems. As we've just read, there are a lot of problems that an older woman can face just because she's a woman. But there are other diseases both men and women over the age of 40 suffer from. Women have to be more careful in monitoring their general health to ensure they're ready to face their toughest decade yet. That begins with knowing what's likely to go wrong with your body and making the necessary dietary and lifestyle changes.

DIABETES

Many Asian women over 40 suffer from Type 2 diabetes. In this disease, the illness and symptoms tend to develop gradually—over weeks or months—because in Type 2 diabetes you still make insulin (unlike in Type 1 diabetes). You develop diabetes because you do not make enough insulin for your body's needs or the cells in your body do not use insulin properly. This is called insulin resistance. The cells in your body become resistant to normal levels of insulin. This means that you need more insulin than you normally make to keep the blood sugar level down. Women over 40 discovered with Type 2 diabetes often suffer from weight problems. Type 2 diabetes accounts for 90 to 95 percent of all diabetes cases.

What are the symptoms?

As the symptoms of Type 2 diabetes tend to develop gradually, you can become used to being thirsty and tired and you may not recognize that you are ill for some time. However, some people with Type 2 diabetes do not have any symptoms if the blood sugar level is not too high. Some common symptoms of Type 2 diabetes are:

Excessive thirst (polydipsia): A woman with diabetes loses the ability to absorb sugar which spills over to the blood stream. This excessive sugar level sends a signal to the brain, which is manifested in the form of being thirsty. Also excess urination may cause the body to lose excess fluid and hence the person feels thirsty. Women who have Type 2 diabetes might instantly discover that they're a lot more hungry and thirsty than normal.

Excessive urination (polyuria): The reason why you make a lot of urine and become thirsty is because glucose leaks into your urine, which pulls out extra water through the kidneys. Increased urination, particularly at night, is a typical sign of Type 2 diabetes.

Fatigue: Women with Type 2 diabetes are a lot more tired than others. It's not uncommon to experience difficulty in getting out of bed in the morning.

Vision problems: Women with Type 2 diabetes may also face difficulty in their vision. Generally, the most reported vision modifications are fuzzy eyesight or double vision. Untreated eye problems caused through diabetes can lead to blindness. You should have regular eye check-ups, especially as you get older, because your eyes can be the early warning signal for many diseases, not just diabetes.

Recurrent infections: Type 2 diabetes can lead to recurrent or chronic vaginal or yeast infections and urinary infections. If you experience excessive itching or soreness in the genital area or yeast infections, it may be a sign of too much sugar in your urine. Additionally, you might notice that it usually takes longer to recover from an infection. Cuts and scratches along with other wounds may also take longer to heal when you have Type 2 diabetes.

Unexplained weight loss and excessive eating: Insufficient insulin in diabetics prevents the body from getting glucose from the blood into the body's cells to use as energy. When this occurs, the body starts burning fat and muscle for energy, causing weight loss.

How is it diagnosed?

A simple dipstick test may detect glucose in a sample of urine. But this is not sufficient to diagnose diabetes. That's why a blood test is needed to make the diagnosis. The blood test detects the level of glucose in your blood. If the blood glucose level is high, it will confirm that you have diabetes. Blood sugars are tested after fasting and then after 2 hours or a glucose tolerance test which measures blood glucose after a measured quantity of glucose can be done. HbA1c or glycosylated haemoglobin is a good test to determine sugar levels over the past 2–3 months. Values below 6 pecent are usually considered normal.

If your blood glucose level is higher than normal over a long period of time, it can gradually damage your blood vessels. This may lead to hardening of the arteries. This can cause problems like angina—chest pain caused by restricted blood supply to the muscles of the heart—and heart attacks. Type 2 diabetes can also cause kidney damage which sometimes develops into kidney failure, eye problems which can affect vision because of the damage to small arteries of the retina at the back of the eye, nerve damage, and foot problems due to poor blood circulation and nerve damage.

How do you treat it?

The best way to treat any type of diabetes is to overhaul your lifestyle. With some minor, dedicated changes, you can actively live with diabetes, even though you will never be cured of it. You can usually reduce the level of your blood glucose if you:

Eat a healthy and balanced diet: Visit a dietician to make changes to your existing diet and switch to a healthy plan. The basic diet is the same as recommended for everyone. The idea that you need special foods if you have diabetes is a myth. Diabetic foods still raise blood glucose levels, contain just as much fat and calories, and are usually more expensive than non-diabetic foods. You should eat a diet low in fat, salt, and sugar, and high in fibre and with plenty of fruit and vegetables.

Do some physical activity regularly: A minimum of 30 minutes of brisk walking at least five times a week is a good way to begin. Anything more vigorous and more often is even better. If walking bores you, swimming, cycling, and dancing are other enjoyable ways to lose weight. Ideally, you should do an activity that gets you at least mildly out of breath and sweaty. Regular physical activity also reduces your risk of having a heart attack.

Lose weight: Getting to a perfect weight is unrealistic for many people. However, losing some weight if you are obese or overweight will help to reduce your blood glucose level. A good side-effect is that you'll feel great about yourself and your body.

HYPERTENSION

Normal blood pressure is 120/80. Hypertension or high blood pressure is common in women in their 40s. It can lead to heart disease, which is the number one cause of death among women. Three out of four women with high blood pressure know they have it. That's the good news because that's a higher percentage than men. The bad news is that less than one out of three is doing anything to control their blood pressure.

Why do most of us ignore this preventable condition? Perhaps it's because traditionally high blood pressure is still thought of as a man's disease. That's partly true. A woman of reproductive age generates sufficient oestrogen to give her some natural defences against high blood pressure. Oestrogen not only allows the blood vessels to remain elastic, it also modulates the behaviour of other hormones which tend to drive up pressure. Until a women reaches menopause, she has a less risk of high blood pressure than a man her own age. However, once a woman passes menopause, the amount of oestrogen her body produces drops significantly. Postmenopausal women have a higher systolic blood pressure (4–5 mmHg) compared with premenopausal or perimenopausal women . Also, the rise in systolic blood pressure per decade was 5 mmHg greater in perimenopausal and postmenopausal women compared with younger women. Because after menopause there is a major decrease in estrogen, it is likely that changes in blood pressure at this stage are due to to this.

Some other causes of hypertension in women are:

Smoking: Cigarette smoking is a major risk factor for high blood pressure.

Salt and potassium: Eating too much salt can increase the risk for developing high blood pressure in some people. Similarly, a diet that is too low in potassium can make the body accumulate too much sodium. Sodium and potassium are important regulators of fluid balance in cells.

Alcohol: Chronic, heavy alcohol use can increase blood pressure. Women are more sensitive than men to the blood pressure effects of alcohol.

Physical inactivity: A sedentary lifestyle can increase the risk of becoming overweight.

Stress: Mental and emotional stress can cause a temporary increase in blood pressure. Chronic stress can lead to engaging in unhealthy behaviours like overeating, smoking, alcohol use, and lack of exercise that contribute to high blood pressure.

Genetics and family history of high blood pressure plays a major role in causing hypertension.

How do I know I have high blood pressure?

Hypertension is a very serious condition and you should be able to first identify it and then seek out ways to treat it. Here are some common symptoms of hypertension.

Feeling tired and confused: Even after having a full night's sleep, you may still feel very sluggish and tired. If tiredness is persistent and you are uncertain about day to day things, it could be a sign of hypertension.

Blurred vision: This is a common sign. If you have sudden blurred vision, it could be hypertension related.

Nose-bleed: Having nose-bleeds are symptom of hypertension.

Irregular heartbeat: This is one of the more serious symptoms of hypertension. If you feel an irregular heartbeat, you should take action and immediately seek help from a doctor.

Blood in urine: Again, this is another sign which could be the result of hypertension.

You can reverse hypertension through a combination of diet and exercise. There are different options such as high blood pressure medication and drugs, or natural cures that can quickly relieve your hypertension and bring you down to a normal range which will eliminate many of the symptoms you have been experiencing.

CHOLESTEROL

Cholesterol is a fatty substance your body needs to rebuild its cells and to make certain hormones. It's carried throughout our body in the bloodstream. Our body only requires a small amount of cholesterol. Too much cholesterol in the bloodstream leads to a condition known as hypercholesterolemia. This is a very common condition, with over half of the world's population suffering from it. Cholesterol levels generally rise with age. High cholesterol can increase your risk of heart disease, stroke, and peripheral vascular disease.

Most of your body's cholesterol—about 80 percent—is

made in the liver. The rest comes from your diet. Dietary cholesterol is found in foods like eggs, meats, and dairy products. The two important types of cholesterol are low-density lipoprotein (LDL) or bad cholesterol, and high-density lipoprotein (HDL) or good cholesterol.

Most of the LDL cholesterol circulates in the blood and remains unused. Normally, the liver removes this extra cholesterol, but many people have more LDL cholesterol than the liver can handle. LDL cholesterol promotes build-up of harmful fatty deposits in the walls of the arteries. HDL is good because it picks up LDL cholesterol from the arteries and tissues and carries it back to the liver, where it can be broken down. Diseases like diabetes, hypothyroidism, liver disease, and kidney disease can raise cholesterol levels.

LDL cholesterol in the bloodstream can settle as fatty deposits on the inside of your blood vessels. These build up over time to become scars, called plaques. LDL cholesterol also stimulates extra cell growth in the lining of the arteries, reducing their diameter. Plaque can clog the arteries. This disease is called atherosclerosis where the arteries harden and can result in chest pain, heart attack, or stroke. High levels of LDL cholesterol cause more plaque build-up and increase the risk of a heart attack.

High cholesterol usually has no obvious symptoms. Like high blood pressure, it's a silent condition that offers no early warning. Most women first discover the problem during a routine blood test and physical examination. They often find they have high blood pressure as well. You can get symptoms from the complications of high cholesterol. These include angina and pain in the calves caused by narrowed arteries to the legs.

High blood cholesterol can lead to dangerous conditions like heart disease. If a woman has blood cholesterol at unsafe levels, she is putting herself at higher risk for these conditions. Women are four times more likely to die from heart disease than breast cancer. This makes reducing heart disease risk factors, like high blood cholesterol, incredibly important. Total blood cholesterol level should be: < 200 mg/dL which is the normal blood cholesterol level, 200–239 mg/dL borderline-high, >240 mg/dL high cholesterol. The desirable LDL level is considered to be less than 100 mg/dL.

What causes high cholesterol?

Much of the blame for high blood cholesterol can be placed on the foods we eat. A diet full of saturated fats can greatly raise a woman's blood cholesterol levels. Genetic factors can also play a role in a woman's risk for high cholesterol, because some women can have high cholesterol levels regardless of how many saturated fats they eat.

What's the best way to beat cholesterol?

A healthy lifestyle is the best defense against high cholesterol. Follow a diet low in saturated fats and cholesterol, eat all sorts of a wide variety of vegetables, whole grains, fruits, nuts, and seeds; boost your level of physical activity; maintain a healthy body weight; and limit your alcohol consumption to no more than two drinks per day. If you quit smoking and keep your blood pressure down, it will help lower your risk of developing angina, heart attack, and stroke.

People who are at a very high risk for coronary artery disease need to be put on medication immediately along with lifestyle changes. Some people think that it's too late to change your habits if you've already had a heart attack. But this is not true. It's vital to reduce your cholesterol to help prevent a second heart attack. Some women with heart disease are now treated with a statin—a drug used to lower high cholesterol levels— even if their cholesterol is normal, especially if their family has a history of high cholesterol. Your body is constantly producing cholesterol, so you must take your medication and follow lifestyle changes to prevent levels from rising.

HYPOTHYROIDISM

A lot of women in their 40s assume that weight gain, fatigue, mood swings, erratic periods, sleep problems, and loss of sex drive is because of perimenopause and menopause. But they don't realize that these can be symptoms of hypothyroidism.

To understand what that means, let's first talk about what the thyroid gland does in your body. Located just under your Adam's apple, your thyroid secretes hormones into the blood stream to control the rate at which every cell and organ turns nutrients into energy. Thyroid hormones control metabolism, growth, body temperature, muscle strength, appetite, and the health of your heart, brain, kidneys, and reproductive system. The thyroid gland responds to the levels of Thyroid Stimulating Hormone (TSH) secreted by the brain's pituitary gland. As the TSH levels in the blood rise, the thyroid responds by making more hormones. As the levels drop, the thyroid is signalled to make less hormones.

If your thyroid doesn't work properly, neither do you. Thyroid disease occurs when your thyroid under- or over-produces the correct amount of thyroid hormone. It can cause elevated cholesterol levels, heart disease, infertility, muscle weakness, osteoporosis, coma, and even death. Thyroid disease can be hereditary.

Why should I worry about hypothyrodism?

Hypothyroidism occurs when the thyroid gland fails to produce enough hormones. Hypothyroidism is most common in women above 40. This disease progresses over time, so the symptoms may not be prominent until you're older. In the first stages of hypothyroidism, you may feel fatigued. Over time your metabolism slows and symptoms become more prominent. These more obvious symptoms are more sensitivity to cold, constipation, pale skin, a bloated face, and high blood cholesterol levels. One of the most common symptoms is inexplicable weight gain. Many women attribute their weight gain to an underactive thyroid, but this is true only in a few cases. You may also suffer from muscle pain and stiffness in your shoulders and hips. Your menstrual cycle may be heavier than normal menstrual cycles. In extreme cases, women even suffer from depression.

How do you fight it?

If you are showing obvious symptoms of hypothyroidism, your doctor will tell you to get a blood test. When the levels of TSH are high and thyroxine is low, it means that you have an underactive thyroid. This is because the pituitary gland is manufacturing more TSH to encourage your thyroid gland to produce more hormones. I have noticed that may doctors, rather than suspecting thyroid problems and getting the proper tests and evaluation, offer women oestrogen and progesterone hormone treatments, antidepressants, or sleeping pills. And women with thyroid problems don't realize that as early as 40, the shifts in oestrogen and progesterone balance—coupled with excess physical and emotional stress in our lives—can make it difficult to keep our thyroid conditions and health in balance. A regular blood test for thyroid is necessary. Treatment is easy, oral tablets taken daily bring thyroid levels to normal very soon.

Goitrogenic foods should be avoided by people with hypothyroidism. These are foods that alter or block iodine absorption. A number of foods are considered goitrogenic and best avoided, including soy products, broccoli, turnips, and cabbage, peanuts and walnuts, mustard, peaches and strawberries, and radishes.

Part 3
Fit at 40

'I'm actually happier with my body now...because the body I have now is the body I've worked for. I have a better relationship with it. From a purely aesthetic point of view, my body was better when I was 22, 23. But I didn't enjoy it. I was too busy comparing it to everyone else's.'

—Cindy Crawford

13

Signs and Symptoms

I'M ALL FOR THE IDEA that 40 is the new 30. But unfortunately, that doesn't change the fact that hitting this number increases the risk of developing certain age-related illnesses. That's why, I cannot emphasize enough the need to be alert for signs and symptoms. But a lot of diseases start out with no signs or symptoms whatsoever.

I was talking to a urologist who had a bypass surgery recently. He said he had no symptoms except for a burning sensation in the throat. He ignored it because he thought it wasn't anything serious. He later said that he never imagined that it would have anything to do with the heart. When the burning wouldn't go away, he decided to take an ECG test, and the result showed that he had suffered a minor heart attack. This is a perfect example of a very irrelevant symptom that can lead to a major problem. I had a patient with a very small growth on the labia. Some women have discolouration in the vulval area or thickening of the skin. The vulva is a neglected area, even among many gynaecologists. But the thickening of the area may turn out to be vulval cancer. It's always better to get yourself tested and rule out a potential problem than ignore it and suffer the consequences later. That's why all women over the age of 40 need to go for regular health check-ups. Every disease has its own indicator. Here are some problems you should look out for.

Vaginal discharge: This is one of the most common problems a woman comes to a gynaecologist with. Thankfully, most women, in my experience, don't neglect it. Vaginal discharge could mean an infection, a sign of pelvic inflammatory disease, an STD, or even cervical cancer. If vaginal discharge is blood-tinged, or if you bleed after intercourse, it's, very often, a sign of cervical cancer.

Urine and stool pattern: You also have to look out for any change in your urinary or stool pattern. If you are passing urine a lot or more often than normal, if you have difficulty in controlling your bladder, if there is incomplete evacuation of urine, you could have a urinary infection or some sort of stone. It could also be a tumour that's pressing upon the urinary bladder. The same things hold true for your stool as well. Are you suddenly getting constipated? Do you have to apply pressure to pass stool? If there is some bleeding while passing stool, you could be suffering from something as simple as haemorrhoids or piles, or it could be a polyp or even cancer of the rectum.

Abdomen pain: Pay attention to any lower abdominal discomfort, pain, cramping, bloating distension, or if you can feel something hard when you touch your abdomen. Lower abdomen discomfort could be a urinary infection, fibroid, or endometriosis. It could even be ovarian cancer. I've spoken about how symptoms of ovarian cancer are acidity or gas. If this persists beyond a few days, it needs to be attended to.

Menstrual cycle shifts: Any change in your menstrual cycle also has to be looked into. As far as gynaecologists go, this is the most important thing to look out for. If you have a 25-day cycle, and suddenly, you start having an 18-day or 35-day cycle, it's a problem. From the time you're 18 till you turn about 40, your period pattern usually stays the same. If you have heavy bleeding, it could suggest fibroids, adenomyosis, thickening of the endometrium and hyperplasia, or cancer. Scanty bleeding is also of relevance because it implies major hormonal change, tuberculosis, or damage to the endometrium. Even the duration of your period cycle is very important. The duration is controlled by the ovary. A great change in the cycle may imply major hormonal changes. Completely erratic bleeding may also imply cancer. Post-menopausal bleeding is the most worrisome situation. Anyone who bleeds one year after menopause should immediately visit a gynaecologist. It doesn't, however, mean that you're suffering from cancer. It can mean drying up of the tissues in your body or atrophy which sometimes can cause a little bleeding.

Weight loss: Any unexplained weight loss or loss of appetite is also not a good sign. It could mean a cancer anywhere in the body. So don't always celebrate weight loss. Similarly, any unexpected weight gain could mean that you're suffering from hypothyroidism. It could also be because of a tumour growing inside your body. A lot of times, women with an abdomen that makes them look 4 or 5 months pregnant come to me. And it turns out to be a large ovarian tumour or fibroid.

Backache: Lower abdomen or pelvic pain, back pain, and pain radiating down to the legs or the back of the buttocks cannot be neglected. A backache could be because a large tumour is pressing across the back of the pelvis. Cervical tumours can manifest as backache. Lower abdominal pain could be pelvic inflammatory disease. Any pain that persists or recurs has to be looked into.

Breast pain: If you find a lump in your breast, it's obvious that you have to get yourself examined. But any heaviness in the breast, pain, sudden increase in size over a short period of time, asymmetry, the look of the skin changing, and discharge from the breast also needs to be immediately attended to. Women with a family history of diseases also have to be very careful, especially for breast and ovarian cancer.

Headaches: Any headache that is unexplained, any fever of unknown origin lasting for more than a couple of days, or any persistent symptom like an irritating cough may not be as simple as a throat infection or allergy. It could be something pressing upon your trachea. A headache with vomiting usually implies nothing. But it could also mean a lesion in the brain or a tumour.

GET THESE TESTS DONE EVERY YEAR

I can't stress enough on the importance of regular health check-ups after you cross 40. Whatever I say in favour of them is inadequate. It's my job to reiterate it every day because I constantly have patients who say that they're fine and that they see no reason to see a doctor. The greatest harm you can do to yourself is not visit the doctor when you're feeling well. The only way you can prevent diseases is by going for regular check-ups. Even though you can't really prevent a disease, you can always pick it up early enough before it turns into a full-blown disease. For instance, diabetes may not show any symptoms till the level of sugar is extremely high. Some patients just feel the urge to drink a lot of water, and would never think of linking it to diabetes. So unless you get yourself tested, you will not know that you're suffering from it. Any uncontrolled diabetes can have an effect on your entire body.

That's why an annual health check-up is the best thing you can do for yourself. Now it's become so much easier because every hospital and laboratory has packages fine-tuned to your individual needs. But these packages sometimes don't offer much because hospitals have to keep the cost low to lure people. There are some packages that don't have a sonography. I find this so ridiculous because a low-cost package without a sonography means that the patient misses out on a check-up of an entire gamut of diseases. So you have to be careful about the packages you choose. Make sure it includes all the important tests.

What should the package have?

- Your package should have cancer screening, pap smear, mammogram, abdominal, and pelvic sonography. It is mandatory to do these tests on an annual basis.
- Every two years, you should get a test for bone density. The test will tell you about the condition of your bones because bones don't deteriorate rapidly.
- There are also blood tests that are not specific to gynaecological issues. We'll ask for a complete blood count (CBC) test and an erythrocyte sedimentation rate (ESR) test which indicates if there is any infection in your body. A lot of times, everything on the test is normal except for the ESR which is very elevated. That needs to

be looked into because there are a lot of infections you can get in our country like tuberculosis which can be a very silent disease.

- Then there is the sugar test, which includes the HbA1C test. It tells you how the sugar levels have been in your body in the last three months.
- There are also the vitamin B12 and D3 tests you should do.
- For some patients, we also recommend the HIV, and Hepatitis B and C tests. Hepatitis B and C may go unnoticed because they are transmitted through the blood and intercourse, and the patient may not have any signs and symptoms. Those two diseases can have a devastating effect on the liver and there have been several instances where patients come to the doctor with complete liver failure and cancer. And upon investigation, it has been found that the patient was suffering from Hepatitis B or C. Even though Hepatitis C is not treatable, we can still keep a close watch on the patient.
- There's also the thyroid stimulating hormone (TSH) test to know how your thyroid gland is doing.
- I'd also recommend a renal and liver function test. They will broadly cover all the tests required for the kidney and liver.
- You also have to test for the prolactin hormone because it can get elevated under different conditions. If the level is high, we can look for a pituitary tumour. Then there is the CA125 test, which is the ovarian tumour marker.

- A lipid profile, which tests for cholesterol, is also important.
- A chest X-ray and ECG should also be on the list.

Recently, a doctor my husband had met on a holiday walked into our clinic. His daughter who is also a doctor had got a job at the Asian Heart Institute in Mumbai and she was required to do a health check-up before joining. The test results showed a massive tumour in her thorax. This is a woman who, from the looks of it, was completely normal and healthy. This shows that the best of us can be blindsided by a disease. A thoracic tumour can be very quiet sometimes and that's probably why she didn't get tested for it. If she had done a chest X-ray, the tumour would have been picked up.

THAT THING CALLED 'STRESS'

I've spoken about all these signs and tests you should do. My intention is not to scare you or turn you into a hypochondriac. This information will help you make better choices for yourself and you will hence lead a life that you're meant to live, reach your full potential without your health dragging you down.

Some of the few things I have learnt since I've entered my 40s is that it's very important to have time to yourself—the time to do things that make you happy. One way I do that is by rising early. It gives me time to exercise or do a bit of yoga.

One other thing I've come to accept as true is the harm that stress does to us. Recently, we had a reunion of our college mates and I met a classmate who is now a top-notch cardiologist in the US. I learnt that he had left his very lucrative practise and had gone back to university for a year because he wanted to learn more. It's not easy for a doctor to do that, but he said that that is what gave him satisfaction and that is what he enjoyed doing. He said that the biggest truth of life is that every problem in our life is related to stress. Stress affects every part of your body, whether it is headache, backache, or cardiac illnesses. Things that you would never connect to stress are related to stress. We're all familiar with the symptoms of stress, but most of us don't know just how harmful it can be. In small doses, it can motivate you to take action, but when stress is excessive or long-lasting it can be dangerous for your physical and mental health. When I say dangerous, I mean depression, cancer, heart attack, premature ageing, anxiety, and much more.

I have another doctor friend who says that most of our problems are psychological. He says that these days he's become more of a counsellor and less of a physician. An orthopaedic doctor friend says that 50 percent of the backaches he sees in women are related to psychological problems. I argued saying that sometimes it is a physical problem, and it's not just in the head. But he wouldn't agree with me. He didn't mean that women are lying about their backs hurting. But the backaches because of stress and anxiety, not because some nerves in the back are damaged. Half of the diseases in the world are related to stress. We know that gastritis, headaches, migraines, and heart attacks are stress related. A few months ago, a 47-year-old urologist was giving a lecture to fellow doctors on a Sunday and collapsed on the dais. He was taken to the hospital, but he passed away. I had met him just a few days before and he was absolutely fine. He was an achiever, very hard working, a perfectionist and because of all this, had no time for himself.

That's why yoga, meditation, destressing, and having some time to yourself is so important. If you met me, you'd think nothing fazes me. But the truth is that I also face a lot of stress. I am severely allergic and we know that allergies are psychosomatic. That's why we need to go beyond what we know of ourselves. When you're young, you get away with a lot of things. But as you grow older, you cannot take your health for granted at all. You have to undo the harm youth has done to you and take hold of your life. I don't mean to say that you give up your partying. But you have to have an overall disciplined life. There is no alternative to that.

14

Exercise

Let's face it. Having a fit body at any age is a challenge. But it only gets more difficult as we get older. After you hit 40, it's very easy to think that you deserve a break from all the running around you've done so far. I wouldn't blame you for thinking like that, especially when I consider the hectic and demanding life we lead. But that attitude won't help.

There are various obvious reasons why a woman gains weight. It doesn't happen overnight. Habits, illnesses, genes, medicines, and emotions are some of the reasons that lead to weight gain. Although you may not be able to control all the factors that lead to gaining weight, you can change your eating and physical activity habits to improve your weight and health.

All the hormonal changes in your body ensure that it's not as fit and supple as it used to be. There is also a lot more water retention now that only adds to your weight. And as you reach 40, your everyday activities start decreasing, but the amount of food you eat remains the same. The Basal Metabolic Rate (BMR) starts falling down. BMR is the rate of energy expended when our bodies are resting. This is the minimum amount of energy needed by the body to perform essential functions like breathing, heartbeat, and blood circulation, etc. If a person's BMR is high, the likelihood that calories from food will be utilized to provide energy rather than being laid down as fat is greater.

THE NEED TO EXERCISE

Women believe that the best way to lose weight is to go on a diet. So some women will eat only fruits while others will have only soups and salads. They cut down on their carbs. Such diets affect their health a lot because what a lot of women don't realize is that the BMR falls further, and they start accumulating more percentage fat. Percentage fat is the amount of fat you have compared to the lean tissue like muscles, bones, body water, organs, etc. Your percentage fat is a clearer indicator of your fitness because regardless of how much you weigh, the higher percentage body fat you have, the more likely you are to develop obesity related diseases like heart disease, high blood pressure, stroke, and type 2 diabetes.

This is why exercise, and more importantly weight training, becomes very important. Women resort to a lot of group exercise classes like spinning and running. But that is only cardio. Your exercise should be a combination of cardio and weight training. Every woman should pick up weights because it increases lean muscle tissue. Lean muscle tissue helps in increasing the BMR. When your percentage fat starts burning, you burn calories faster, even when you rest. Weight train will give you a toned body. I have also observed that women are scared to weight train because they believe they will build big muscles like men. But that will not happen because men and women have different hormones. A woman who has always been thin may put on weight in the abdomen area, hips, and thighs as she enters the 40s. As I said before, diet will not help because you will put on all the weight you had lost as soon as you go off it. Human nature dictates that you will eat double of whatever food you have denied yourself. So the moment you go off a diet, you eat a lot and then you'll put on double the amount of weight and double of amount of percentage fat. That's why the ideal scenario is a balanced diet and exercise with a combination of weight training and cardio.

Also, weight training will ensure that you delay the onset of osteoporosis. It makes your bones dense and it improves your HDL:LDL cholesterol ratio so that your lipid profile changes. It doesn't matter how much cardio you do; you have to take up weight training. A lot of women in their 40s ask me why they should go for weight training at their age. In fact, it becomes more important at 40. Your lean muscle tissue has to increase, your BMR has to go up, and your percentage fat has to go down. Remember that muscle is youth. Weight training will give shape to your body.

MY TIPS TO HAVE A FAB BODY

It is a myth that certain exercises are for men and certain exercises are only for women. All exercises are for everyone. Men and women both want good shoulders, thin waist, good butt, good legs, and good arms. These are some of the ways by which you can achieve that.

- Do not try fad diets. Don't go online and download some diet for yourself. In the long run, all these diets have harmful effects on your body because you don't know how they affect your liver and kidneys and make them do extra work. High-protein diets are also very harmful because they cause an extra load on the kidneys.
- What suits one woman may not suit you. That is true for both exercise and diet.
- Get a fitness assessment done. It will tell you your BMR, percentage fat, muscle strength and endurance, abdomen strength, flexibility, cardio respiratory endurance, grip strength, and psychological analysis. My gym is the only one in the entire country which does this. At the end of your assessment, your trainer gets a graph of your body, which helps them chart a suitable exercise plan for you.
- Ensure that you have a customized exercise plan and diet.
- Concentrate on natural foods and a balanced diet.

- A lot of women complain of bloating, especially by the end of the day. Less water intake is a common reason. Dehydration causes bloating, so drink lots of water. Bloating can also be caused by PMS, which is very different at 40 than when you were younger.
- You can also suffer from an undetected gluten allergy or you may be lactose intolerant. It's important to get these food allergies tested. Once you know that you have a particular allergy, you can avoid those foods by going to a proper dietician. Don't make your own diet chart. Dieticians who tell you to not to weight train are giving the wrong advice.
- Include a lot of flax seeds, omega 3 and 6 fatty acids, three portions of fruits, and lots of raw vegetables and salads in your diet. The more colourful your veggies and salads, the more antioxidants they have.

Be active, be active, be active

I cannot stress this enough. I know so many women in their 40s who just sit around and don't move a muscle. Your general activity quotient has to increase. Use the stairs, answer the doorbell, get that glass of water on your own. Small changes like these make a huge difference. If you have a desk job, walk every two hours. Whatever happens, exercise. It doesn't matter if it's raining outside or it's a hot day. You have to exercise.

One problem that I encounter among housewives of

this age is that because their kids have grown up and the husband is busy with work, they find a void in their lives. They suddenly have nothing to do. That's never a good state of being. So get your mind involved for psychological balance. Everyone is so focused on physical well-being that the mental aspect is ignored. Mental fitness is also very important. If you have nothing to do, pick up a hobby, learn a musical instrument, join an NGO, or start something of your own. It's never too late to do all these things. Life is not all about your husband and your kids. You have to think about yourself also.

Going to the gym is like a one-hour appointment with yourself. You go to the parlour for facials and to groom your body. But if you exercise, your hair and skin will automatically be good. Exercising will give you good posture and a positive attitude. It will release chemicals like endorphins that will make you feel happy. It will build your confidence and self-esteem and you will look at problems with a positive attitude. Your life gets very disciplined because of your exercise schedule. Your eating habits will be monitored because your gym time is monitored. And because of your lifestyle, even your house gets disciplined. Exercise is like preventive medicine. When you exercise, your cholesterol and blood pressure is maintained. Your heart becomes strong. A lot of women at this age complain of knee problems, but with exercise, your injuries are reduced. Women keep rubbing balms and popping pills, but if you exercise regularly, you will not need all these things. Remember, being fit is sexy.

Your body is waiting for a challenge. If you pick up 5 pounds during weight training today, the next week your body will want more. If you're running for 5 km today, your body will want to be pushed to 7 km the next day. You are the one decaying your body. Just like you send your car for preventive maintenance, your body will break down if you don't give it the preventive medicine of exercise. It is the best anti-ageing medicine.

15
Diet

IF YOU'VE CROSSED THE AGE of 40, you've probably noticed that it's become a lot easier to gain a few kilos than to lose them. The foods that you ate without care in your 20s and 30s, now stick to your body like glue, adding bulk to your midsection. Research shows that when combined with a little regular exercise, what you eat and when you eat it are your metabolic secret weapons for building muscle mass, the body's prime calorie-burning tissue, and a key driver of your metabolism. That's why it is so important to safeguard muscle mass and turn up the heat on your body's natural calorie-frying furnace.

To start with, you have to eat healthy, especially foods that are rich in protein and fibre. That's because they support calorie-burning muscle mass. Next, you should strength-train twice a week to fight muscle loss. While doing that, you should also squeeze in a quick cardio workout 5 times a week to hike all day calorie-burn.

Just because you have hit menopause doesn't mean that your life is over. Menopause can most certainly be a positive time of your life. Although menopause can cause some noticeable and uncomfortable changes, these can be effectively managed with diet and exercise. Understanding what's really going on in our bodies can help us find natural solutions to the health challenges this phase of life brings us. Because oestrogen levels decrease, our risk of heart disease and osteoporosis increases. Menopause is also linked to high blood pressure and weight gain, as well as a higher risk for breast cancer. While hormone replacement therapy can help, we can also battle these negative forces with proper nutrition.

Peimenopause and menopause is a time in your life when eating gets tricky. Although we seem to be endlessly conscious of what we eat, what we weigh, and how we look, menopause brings special attention to the importance of a healthy diet. Add to that, a slowing metabolism and health risks that rise with age, it's clear that we have to make every calorie count for something good. How do we set priorities in the face of all these competing needs? We want to stay healthy, look good, and yet not overdo it.

Every woman experiences different symptoms of menopause. Some women have hot flashes while others feel irritable. A smaller number of women battle headaches, nausea, or night sweats. Whatever your symptoms, these food strategies might help make your years around menopause a little more comfortable. They'll help you manage your menopause symptoms while also protecting your heart and your bones. Remember that what works for one woman may not work for another, and what works for you now may not work a year later.

This is a 9-point plan that I tell every patient who comes to me:

Eat more tofu and soya: Soya is said to give relief from hot flashes. Although that benefit is still being debated by researchers, we do know that soya helps protect our heart and arteries by lowering bad cholesterol. Choose tofu dishes instead of meat at your local Chinese restaurant Make fruit smoothies with soya protein powder. Drink chocolate or plain soya milk. Buy baked tofu at the supermarket and experiment making dishes at home. Add it to salads or stir-fry it with veggies. Even try it on crackers. Buy canned soya beans and add them to soups.

Eat more fruits and vegetables: Foods with boron and phytoestrogens ease menopause symptoms. Boron increases the body's ability to hold on to oestrogen. It also helps keep our bones strong by decreasing the amount of calcium we excrete each day. The top sources of boron that also contain phytoestrogens are plums, prunes, strawberries, apples, tomatoes, pears, grapes, grapefruit, oranges, asparagus, beetroots, bell peppers, broccoli stems, cabbage, cauliflower, carrots, cucumbers, lettuce, onions, soya beans, and sweet potatoes.

Eat beans a lot more often than you usually do: Beans are a nutritionally efficient food because they offer so many health benefits in one little package. They slow the absorption of glucose in the bloodstream, thus curbing your appetite longer. They're full of fibre, contain phytoestrogens, are a low-fat source of protein, and are also a good source of many vitamins and minerals, including calcium, folic acid, and vitamin B-6.

Choose your beverages wisely: Women experiencing symptoms of menopause may have trouble sleeping well along with hot flashes. Caffeine can make you both moody and even more tired, since it interferes with sleep, especially if you drink it in the afternoon. The other problem with caffeine is that we rarely drink it alone. Since we add sugar or cream, we make the drink even less healthy. Try herbal peppermint tea for a gentle pick-me-up on a menopause diet.

Be a grazer, not a gorger: Compared with people who gorge on a few big meals a day, grazers, who eat frequent mini meals, have steadier moods, are less likely to develop diabetes, have a healthier immune system, tend to be leaner, enjoy lower blood cholesterol, and levels of stress hormones.

Eat calcium-rich food every day: Although we believe that we should get the bulk of our nutrients from the foods we eat, most women, especially those watching their weight (hence, cutting back on calories), often don't get enough calcium or vitamin D in their daily diets. After menopause, women should aim to get 1200 milligrams of calcium daily. Research shows that calcium and vitamin D helps keep bones strong. In one study, postmenopausal women who took calcium and vitamin D supplements regularly had fewer hip fractures. Calcium and vitamin D also help with weight management, possibly stimulating the breakdown of fat cells and suppressing the development of new ones.

Calcium-rich foods you should try to work into your diet are low-fat yoghurt, low-fat milk, calcium-fortified orange juice, broccoli, and firm tofu. If you're not getting enough calcium from food, talk to your doctor about a supplement that contains calcium and vitamin D, as vitamin D helps you absorb calcium.

Avoid high-sugar foods: The problem with sugar is that it makes the skin lose the plump, elastic qualities that underlie a youthful appearance. What happens is that sugar attaches itself to any protein in the body and produces harmful molecules called 'advanced glycation end products'. These reduce the effectiveness of elastin and collagen—proteins in the skin that help maintain its youthful appearance.

Add flaxseeds to your diet: Flaxseeds have been proven to reduce hot flashes. In one study, women consumed four tablespoons of ground flaxseeds daily—two in the morning, two in the evening. After six weeks, the frequency of their hot flashes dropped. Researchers believe the lingams in flax offer a natural, less potent oestrogen effect on hot flashes than synthetic hormone therapy. Flaxseeds are also one of the best plant sources of omega 3 fatty acids and they provide both soluble fibre, linked to reduced risk of heart disease, and insoluble fibre, which provides valuable roughage. But for your body to absorb the benefits, the seeds must be ground.

Exercise. Exercise. Exercise: Exercise helps prevent diseases, improves your stamina, strengthens and tones your body, keeps your weight under control, and improves the overall quality of life. Need I say more?

Foods that cure

At this time of life, many women still take their good health for granted, and healthy eating and exercise are often put on the back burner. But as we grow older, good nutrition and regular exercise becomes even more important. After the age of 40, the metabolic rate (the speed at which the body burns calories) drops, but the drop is very modest, and the real reason many people in this age bracket start to suffer from middle-aged spread is lack of exercise. Excess weight, particularly around the middle, is a risk factor for heart disease, diabetes, and osteoarthritis, and the longer you wait before you tackle the problem, the harder it becomes.

A diet rich in antioxidants will help protect against problems like heart disease, Alzheimer's, and certain types of cancer. Despite an overall good diet, there are certain foods that help women tackle problems that are known to crop up in the 40s.

INSOMNIA AND HEADACHES

Studies suggest that eating carbs can increase the release of tryptophan, an amino acid that helps the brain manufacture serotonin. This helps people fall asleep.

Say yes to:

- Eating a piece of toasted whole grain bread before going to bed.
- Egg whites and warm milk.
- Cherries contain melatonin, a substance found in the body, which helps regulate sleep.
- 3 dates before sleep with 1 cup of skimmed milk.

Say no to:

- Large meals. When you eat a large meal, digestion brings blood into the abdomen, raises body temperature, and tells the hypothalamus in the brain to send a signal that causes hot flashes. Eating smaller meals can help reduce hot flashes.

- Caffeine. Coffee, tea, colas, and dark chocolate contain caffeine. They may trigger hot flashes and affect your sleep. Drink water instead, especially in the late afternoon and evenings.

Bloating

During the menopause transition, another common symptom is bloating, which may be due to hormone fluctuations, overproduction of estradiol, and conversion of androgen (a male hormone) to oestrogen through a process called aromatization, which increases with age and body weight.

Say yes to:

- Foods and herbs that have diuretic properties, such as celery seeds, parsley, berries, asparagus, artichokes, melon, and watercress. And drink plenty of water and herbal teas.
- One to two litres of lukewarm water every day.

Say no to:

- Sugary and high-sodium foods such as frozen dinners and canned soups should be avoided. Read the sugar and sodium content on food labels, and reduce the amount of sugar and salt that you add to foods and beverages.

MOOD SWINGS

During the transition to menopause, many women report a decreased sense of well-being due to irritability and mood swings. Good nutrition plays a major role in setting your mood right.

Say yes to:

- Eating vegetable such as asparagus, Brussels sprouts, and beetroot, which are rich in B vitamins. Green vegetables such as spinach and peas are high in folic acid, a member of the B-complex group that also helps stabilize your mood because it's needed to make serotonin.

Say no to:

- Sugary foods, which cause a rise in blood sugar and increase mood disturbances.

IRRITABILITY

Women get irritated because they feel low, are tired most of the time, and suffer from the 'poor me' syndrome. At this time, what they crave the most is sugar.

Say yes to:

- Having sugar in the indirect form. This includes coconut water and dryfruit milkshakes.
- Figs, fruit yoghurts.

- Chana-gud is also great. Chana provides the iron and gud the sugar, so this is a great snack.

Say no to:

- Ice cream, chocolates that have very high sugar content. All deep-fried food.

MEMORY LAPSES

These usually happen in women over 40 because of loss of concentration and anxiety. Studies have found that brain functioning showed evidence of decline in memory, reasoning, and comprehension as early as age 45.

Say yes to:

- Fish, chicken, egg whites, curd, sprouts, especially moong, and wheat atta.
- Vitamin B-complex supplements.

Say no to:

- Foods with high sugar content like sweets and chocolates.
- All white food like pasta, noodles, bread, and rice.

EATING BETTER

If your 40th birthday has come and gone, chances are that you've seen some changes in your body composition. The 40s are when hormonal changes begin, and those changes are known to slow down your metabolic rate, causing the body to burn calories less efficiently. That means that the same diet that kept you slim and healthy in your 20s and 30s may promote weight gain. That is one of the most common symptoms of perimenopause. However, midlife weight gain is not inevitable. Changing the way you eat can help you gain the upper hand against middle-age spread.

Before beginning a new diet or exercise routine to help with the symptoms and changes of menopause, it is important to discuss your condition, and how to safely modify your lifestyle with a medical professional.

16

Anti-ageing

WHETHER CONSCIOUSLY OR NOT, WE associate age and attractiveness of a woman with the appearance of her skin. Like other organs of the body, the physiological functions and structures within the skin continuously decline with advancing age. Dry skin, fine lines and deep wrinkles, enlarged pores, and age spots are all outward signs we associate with ageing skin. Learning more about the process of skin ageing can help you understand how to delay and minimize some skin ageing processes.

Just like machines and engines, our body too ages because of the cumulative damages to our cells, tissues, and organs that exceeds our body's ability to repair them. These damages lead to obvious signs of ageing: sags, bulges, and wrinkles.

WHAT ARE THE CAUSES OF SKIN AGEING?

Research shows that there are two distinct types of ageing. Ageing caused by the genes we inherit is called intrinsic or natural ageing. The other type of ageing is extrinsic or external ageing and is caused by environmental factors, such as exposure to the sun's rays.

INTRINSIC AGEING

Intrinsic ageing, also known as the natural ageing process, is a continuous process that normally begins in our mid-20s. Within the skin, collagen production slows down, and elastin, the substance that enables the skin to snap back into place, has a bit less spring. Dead skin cells do not shed as quickly and the turnover of new skin cells decreases slightly.

The signs of natural ageing are:

- Fine wrinkles.
- Thin and transparent skin.
- Loss of underlying fat, leading to hollowed cheeks and eye sockets as well as noticeable loss of firmness on the hands and neck.
- Bones that shrink away from the skin due to bone loss, which causes sagging skin.
- Dry skin that may itch.
- Inability to sweat sufficiently to cool the skin.
- Greying hair that eventually turns white.

- Hair loss.
- Unwanted hair.

EXTRINSIC AGEING

A number of extrinsic or external factors often act together with the normal ageing process to prematurely age our skin. Most premature ageing is caused by sun exposure. Other external factors that prematurely age our skin are repetitive facial expressions, gravity, sleeping positions, and smoking. Let's discuss how each damages the skin.

The sun

Without protection from the sun's rays, just a few minutes of exposure each day over the years can cause noticeable changes to the skin.

Freckles, age spots, spider veins on the face, rough and leathery skin, fine wrinkles that disappear when stretched, loose skin, a blotchy complexion, actinic keratoses (thick, wart-like, rough, reddish patches of skin), and skin cancer can all be traced to sun exposure. With repeated exposure to the sun, the skin loses the ability to repair itself, and the damage accumulates. Several scientific studies have shown that repeated exposure to ultra-violet (UV) rays breaks down collagen and impairs the synthesis of new collagen. The sun also attacks our elastin. The skin then becomes loose, wrinkled, and leathery much earlier with unprotected exposure to sunlight.

Facial expressions

Repetitive facial movements actually lead to fine lines and wrinkles. Each time we use a facial muscle, a groove forms beneath the surface of the skin, which is why we see lines form with each facial expression. As skin ages and loses its elasticity, the skin stops springing back to its line-free state, and these grooves become permanently etched on the face as fine lines and wrinkles.

Gravity

Gravity constantly pulls on our bodies. Changes related to gravity become more pronounced as we age. Gravity causes the tip of the nose to droop, the ears to elongate, eyelids to fall, sagging jowls (lower part of a person's cheek), and the upper lip to disappear while the lower lip becomes more pronounced.

Sleeping positions

Resting your face on the pillow in the same way every night for years on end also leads to wrinkles. Called sleep lines, these wrinkles eventually become etched on the surface of the skin. Women who tend to sleep on their side are most likely to see these lines appear on their chin and cheeks.

Smoking

Cigarette smoking causes biochemical changes in our bodies that accelerate ageing. Research shows that a person who smokes 10 or more cigarettes a day for a minimum of 10 years is statistically more likely to develop deeply wrinkled, leathery skin than a non-smoker.

HOW DO YOU PREVENT THE PROCESS OF AGEING?

While you cannot stop or even slow down the natural ageing process, you can take some steps to ensure that signs of premature ageing don't show on your face. This mostly means effective protection from the sun.

- Stay out of the sun between 10 am and 4 pm, when the sun's rays are the strongest.
- Wear protective clothing like long sleeves and use an umbrella when you're outdoors during the day.
- Apply sunscreen every day throughout the year regardless of the season. Sunscreen should offer UVA and UVB protection and have a Sun Protection Factor (SPF) of 15 or higher. Sunscreen should be applied 20 minutes before going outdoors to every part of your skin that will be exposed. Reapply if you've been sweating.

Hyperpigmentation

Hyperpigmentation or melasma or chloasma is characterized by tan or brown patches on the cheeks, nose, forehead, and chin. This condition is extremely common in women. Sometimes dark patches develop on a woman's face during pregnancy. This is known as the mask of pregnancy or chloasma, and it usually fades after delivery.

What causes hyperpigmentation?

Despite a lot of research, the cause of chloasma is not totally known. But many doctors believe that increased levels of pregnancy hormones cause the pigment-producing cells in the skin called melanocytes to produce more pigment. Although it can affect anyone, hyperpigmentation is particularly common in pregnant women and those who are taking oral contraceptives or hormone replacement therapy.

Dark, irregular patches commonly found on the upper cheek, nose, lips, and forehead are common symptoms of hyperpigmentation. These patches develop gradually over time. Hyperpigmentation does not cause any other symptoms beyond cosmetic discolouration.

Women with light brown skin are particularly susceptible to developing hyperpigmentation. Genetic predisposition is also a major factor in determining whether a woman will develop hyperpigmentation or not. The incidence also increases in women with a thyroid problem. In rare cases, it is also caused by allergic reaction to medications and cosmetics.

How can it be treated?

Hyperpigmentation requires a doctor's attention and treatment differs from woman to woman. But usually, most patients get face treatments with AHA packs and skin lightning creams as well as sessions with microcurrent machines, microdermabrasion, chemical peel, and laser surfacing. While I will explain these procedures in detail later, here's a gist of what they're all about.

Microcurrent involves a machine that passes current of negligible voltage on the superficial facial skin. This makes the facial skin undergo a sort of mini workout and it triggers an increase in the amount of blood circulation in the facial area, thus aiding in quicker removal of toxins. Microcurrent therapy for the face also causes exfoliation of skin, which removes superficial dead cells and reveals the newer and healthier cells.

Microdermabrasion is an electronic form of mechanical exfoliation that uses micro-crystals or crushed diamonds to essentially 'sand' the surface of the skin. It also utilizes strong suction which helps remove even more dead cells and debris. The suction also gives a temporary plumping effect to the skin and helps remove pigmentation.

A chemical peel is a skin resurfacing procedure in which a chemical solution is applied to the skin to peel away the top layers. The skin that grows back after a chemical peel is smoother and younger looking.

Laser resurfacing is a treatment to reduce facial wrinkles and skin irregularities such as blemishes or acne scars. The technique directs short, concentrated pulsating beams of light at irregular skin, precisely removing the skin layer by layer.

While these are professional treatments, you can also try some home remedies to dull the effects of hyperpigmentation. Firstly, start by using sunscreen because sunlight will worsen your condition. Use cool clothes and apply ice on sunburned areas. Applying soothing lotions that contain aloe vera also help. But do not use creams unless your doctor tells you to.

What treatments do dermatologists offer to fight ageing?

If you are bothered by visible signs of ageing, a number of treatments are available.

Facial rejuvenation

All over the world, people spend huge amounts of money each year on skin-care products that promise to erase wrinkles, lighten age spots, and eliminate itching, flaking, or redness. But the simplest and cheapest way to keep your skin healthy and young looking is to stay out of the sun.

Sunlight is a major cause of the skin changes we think of as ageing, changes such as wrinkles, dryness, and age spots. As your skin ages, it becomes thinner and loses fat, so it looks less plump and smooth, and veins and bones in particular become more prominent.

That's why women consider facial skin rejuvenation. Your appearance greatly affects how you and others feel about you. It is, therefore, perfectly natural for older women who feel young and healthy to want their skin to reflect their mental space. Facial rejuvenation can effectively reduce wrinkles, treat sun spots, tighten loose skin, improve skin tone and colour, remove blotchiness, and eliminate damaged blood vessels. Thousands of women undergo some form of facial skin rejuvenation every year.

Great strides in surgical techniques and technology enable dermatologists to achieve subtle, effective results. Today, procedures are safer and less invasive, allowing patients to heal more quickly than ever before. This means little or no downtime. Treatment is usually performed in a dermatologist's office, which offers the patient a convenient and cost-effective option for treating signs of ageing.

Facial rejuvenation treatment differs depending on the damage on your skin. For minimal amounts of ageing and skin damage, dermatologists ideally do chemical peels, fillers, Botulinum rejuvenation, non-ablative lasers, and microdermabrasion. For moderate and severe amounts of ageing and skin damage, I'd add dermabrasion Erbium-

YAG laser Coblation, fractional resurfacing photodynamic therapy, and CO2 laser tumescent liposuction.

Autologous fat transplant

Autologous fat (one's own fat) transfer is today's No. 1 filling agent for loss of volume and creases on our faces. As we age, the appearance of creases on our face is inevitable. Even though these creases are a part of the normal ageing process and there is nothing we can do to stop it, we can fill out the creases with fat, thus making them decrease or appear less prominent. As we get older, we start to lose fat from our upper face. This loss of fat and associated loose skin starts to show up in the cheek area, giving us a sad, gloomy look. By placing fat in the upper region of our face, we produce an uplift effect. This reshapes our face to look more youthful.

As well as losing volume from the face, the backs of the hands can also loose volume. That's why autologous fat is the ideal filler to rejuvenate the back of the hands, as well as the nasal labial fold (mouth to nose grooves) or any other depression of the body.

Since it is the patient's own fat, there is no risk of rejection and no possibility of an allergic reaction. This procedure is mainly used to produce a more youthful look and for recontouring of the face, hands, and other body contours. Fat transfer to the face is a safe, natural, non-allergenic procedure. With fat transfer, it is possible to have fat removed from your thighs using liposuction, for example, and then transferred to any area of your body. Reinjected fat lasts longer in larger areas of the body that don't move as much, like the face, so it is very successful for the correction of sunken cheeks, because this area does not move as often. Fat transfer can also correct ageing of the hands, and post-surgical and post-traumatic defects. But not every area of the body responds well to fat transfer. The breasts, for instance, are not appropriate for it.

How is the procedure performed?

Fat transfer is performed on an outpatient basis. Both the area from which the fat is taken and the treatment site are anesthetized. Using a small needle attached to a syringe, fat is removed from a donor site, where the fat is most tightly packed, such as the abdomen or the buttocks. Once removed, the fat is processed to remove excess fluids, and then reinjected using another needle, which is placed under the skin, beneath the wrinkle. The amount of fat put in each area is always more than needed. That's because we know that initially about 40 percent to 50 percent will be absorbed by the body. The rest will stay. We always keep some of the patient's fat in our fat bank freezer. So, if in the future you need more rejuvenation on a particular area, we already have the fat ready. Most patients need around two to three sessions, but by having the fat stored in our fat bank, there is no need to harvest it again. Pathological studies have shown that we can use the fat for up to two years after harvesting. The cells of the fat tissue maintain all their anatomical and physiological properties for this duration. Harvesting the fat cells for reinjection is often performed with other procedures such as liposuction, tummy tuck, or cosmetic breast surgery. When fat is harvested during another procedure, it is often possible to obtain a larger amount of fat, and then freeze and store it for future use.

Are there any complications?

When performed by a qualified surgeon, complications from a fat transplant are infrequent and usually minor. Nevertheless, there is always a possibility of complications, including reaction to the anaesthesia, infection, and haematoma (bleeding under the skin). This can result in increased bruising, temporary swelling, and a slight asymmetry in healing or scarring.

Botox and fillers

Botox is a toxin that is used for temporary removal of facial wrinkles. Repeated muscular contractions such as frowning and squinting form lines known as dynamic wrinkles. Botox works by relaxing the muscles that cause dynamic wrinkles, giving the face a more relaxed and refreshed appearance. The procedure is so simple and quick that patients can often have it done during their lunch hour.

It is now the fastest growing cosmetic procedure used by hundreds of thousands of women worldwide who want to take control of their appearance and look as good as they feel. Botox is now also widely used for excessive sweating in underarms, as well as on palms and soles.

IS BOTOX DANGEROUS?

Botox, when administered by a trained doctor, takes just a few minutes. The wrinkle-smoothing result can be seen within days, and can last for upto 10 to 12 months. It's a simple and non-invasive treatment. Today, thousands of patients have discovered the beauty of Botox injections in helping them looking as good as they feel.

Microdermabrasion

Microdermabrasion is a non-invasive treatment that propels natural mineral crystals on to the surface of the skin for gentle epidermal abrasion that reveals newer, healthier, younger skin.

Microdermabrasion works in two ways:

Correction: The speed of the crystal flow causes an abrasive action that gently removes the surface layers of the skin, allowing smoother, fresher skin to emerge.

Stimulation: The vacuum action helps stimulate microcirculation, increasing the blood supply that provides nutrients needed for skin regeneration. It also stimulates formation of new collagen and elastin to improve skin texture and elasticity.

Is it painful?

The treatment is performed with little discomfort. At the most, sensitive patients might experience a slight sensation like light sunburn. After treatment, the skin has a pink glow, and you can resume your normal activities almost immediately.

Rejuvenating neck and chest skin

With age, many women experience more and more pronounced skin blotchiness and spider veins, called telangiectasias (visible veins on face), on the sides of the neck and chest.

The neck and the chest are particularly prone to these white indentations because of the thinning skin in the area. Chemical peels and bleaching agents applied directly to the skin help with the pigmentation problems, including white and brown spots. Laser and light treatments, including pulsed light lasers, reduce redness. Laser procedures and chemical peels can lighten the skin. As a result, dermatologists can also lighten those areas, such as the neck, which can contrast the face, with a trichloracetic acid (TCA) peel. This helps to blend in the areas so that the face doesn't look strikingly lighter than the neck and chest.

Non-ablative lasers are tools dermatologists use to treat sun damage on the neck and chest area. While lasers work by heating and removing the top skin layers, non-ablative lasers work beneath the skin's surface by targeting cells that absorb the light's energy. The underlying sources of the skin discolouration break apart from the laser's light and become absorbed in the body. After a series of non-ablative laser treatments, dermatologists can reduce the signs of ageing and sun damage, including fine wrinkles, freckles and irregular pigmentation, especially on the face, neck, and chest. Women who have these procedures can return immediately to activities because non-ablative laser therapy causes no downtime.

How can your hands look younger?

Many women focus on rejuvenating the skin on their faces but forget about their ageing hands. Among the most common problems associated with ageing hands are wrinkles and brown spots, which respond to a number of treatments. If you don't want to undergo any procedures, there is the option of dermatologist prescribed bleaching creams, which you can rub on your hands on a regular basis. These work subtly to reduce the discolouration of dark pigmented spots.

But if you want faster, better results, chemical peels, from the superficial glycolic acid to the medium TCA peels which work to remove dead skin cells and stimulate the production of new skin cells, are the way to go.

Some dermatologists also use lasers like the Q-switched Nd: YAG laser, to change the hands' skin colour and remove spots. Unlike the face, hands are much easier to treat. Typically, laser treatments correcting discolourations on the hands take about 10 minutes in a dermatologist's office.

The skin on the hands also tends to be thin. Dermatologists have the option of using fat transplantation from other areas of the body to give the hands a more youthful plumpness. This can be done in conjunction with other procedures to lighten the dark areas on the hands.

What about the legs?

Varicose and spider veins on the legs can worsen with age. Here too dermatologists have an arsenal of treatments to bring youthfulness back to the skin on the legs.

Varicose veins are abnormally swollen or enlarged blood vessels caused by a weakening of the vein's walls. Dermatologists can treat the condition with a procedure called radio frequency closure. This involves inserting a small tube, or catheter, into the varicose vein through a small puncture. The catheter delivers radio frequency energy to the vein wall, causing it to shrink and seal shut. Patients generally do not feel pain during the procedure and often can return immediately afterwards to activities.

Dermatologists today treat leg spider veins with lasers, which were traditionally reserved for the face. Newer versions of laser technology, including the Nd: YAG 1064nm, use wavelengths to penetrate the skin of the legs without heating the pigment. This reduces the risk of burning or injury to the skin. Typically, two to five treatments, which last about 15 minutes each, are required to remove spider veins.

The mainstay of leg vein treatments continues to be injection with sclerosing solutions or sclerotherapy, a method in which the solution is injected with a very fine needle directly into the blood vessel.

If you're considering injectables...

As we age, our faces begin to show the effects of gravity, sun exposure, and years of facial muscle movement, such as smiling, chewing, and squinting. The underlying tissues that keep our skin looking youthful and plumped up begin to break down, often leaving laugh lines, smile lines, crow's feet, or facial creases over the areas where this muscle movement occurs.

Soft-tissue fillers, most commonly called injectable collagen or fat, can help fill in these lines and creases, temporarily bringing back your smoother, more youthful-looking appearance. When injected beneath the skin, these fillers plump up creased and sunken areas of the face. They can also add fullness to the lips and cheeks. Injectable fillers can be used alone or along with a resurfacing procedure, such as a laser treatment, or a recontouring procedure, such as a facelift.

Know your options

Injected collagen and fat are primarily used to improve the appearance of the skin's texture. They can help fill out deep facial wrinkles, creases and furrows, sunken cheeks, skin depressions, and some types of scars. They can also be used to add a fuller, more sensuous look to the lips. Injectables are usually not sufficient for severe surface wrinkles on the face such as multiple vertical 'lipstick lines' that sometimes form around the mouth. Instead, your doctor may suggest a resurfacing technique such as chemical peel, dermabrasion, or laser treatments. Rather than filling in facial lines, resurfacing methods strip away the outer layers of the skin to produce a smoother appearance.

Deep folds in the face or brow caused by overactive muscles or by loose skin can be treated better with cosmetic surgery, such as a facelift or browlift. Injectables are sometimes used in conjunction with facial surgery procedures. However, injectables alone cannot change facial contours the way surgery can.

Keep in mind that a plastic surgeon is a specialist that can offer you the full gamut of the most advanced treatments ranging from cosmetic surgery, refinishing techniques, laser therapy, injectables, and the use of other fillers. You have to work alongside your surgeon to determine what procedure or a combination of procedures is the best choice for you.

Fortunately, you can turn back the clock on your skin. Even if you did not properly care for your skin in the years gone by, there are many technologically advanced procedures that help repair sun damage and reverse some of the effects of both biological and mechanical ageing. Because youthful, healthy skin portrays confidence and beauty, we are all concerned with what we assume is inevitable skin ageing. The good news is that we have more control than we realize over the rate at which our skin ages.

Conclusion

THIS BOOK IS A CONVERSATION I'd love to have with every woman over the age of 40. Since that's nearly impossible, I wrote this book—so that every woman has all the information she needs to take care of herself.

In all my years as a gynaecologist, the most important thing I've learned is that there's no alternative to getting yourself screened and tested for potential diseases. Regular visits to the doctor will assess risk of future medical problems. It also encourages a healthy lifestyle. Your health is all about nipping the problem in the bud before it becomes a major issue.

In my experience, every woman says that she feels healthy and doesn't have a problem. But do not take your health for granted. That, I think, is the most important message of this book. Even if you are feeling completely well and healthy and everything is going fine in your life, you need to get checked. You will be shocked by the number of people—men and women—who find out that they have a disease when they start investigating their body further. You have to find time for yourself, no matter how busy you are. There will be days when you'll binge and behave badly, and that's fine. What's life if you don't forget your worries once in a while and just have fun? But you also have to remember that there is no replacement for a disciplined lifestyle. You have to be careful about what you subject your body to. If you know that something's wrong and that you can prevent it, you owe it to yourself to try every means possible to protect yourself and your body. There is nothing better than preventive action because once you have a disease, it is already too late.

Life-threatening diseases can happen to the best of us. But it's possible to live with a serious disease like diabetes, all because you caught the disease at the right time.

Your 40s are considered a mid-point, the top of the hill. It's a big milestone, but you've still got miles to go. Don't let body changes and health hazards send you downhill. Some of the factors that affect your health are out of our control, like your family's medical legacy. If your mother or sister have had breast cancer, you might be more likely to have breast cancer too. But you can control the lifestyle choices you make. And these choices either enrich or endanger the quality of your health. What sort of foods you eat, and how much physical activity you fit into your life, may make or break your health. As Oprah Winfrey said, 'There are no back doors, no free rides [to fitness]. There's just you, this moment, and a choice.'

Good health is a combination of factors like your mind, body, and emotions. I wanted to focus on each of them and realized that they are all interlinked. The way you look and feel also contributes to the feeling of well-being. Never forget that wellness is not just absence of disease; it's the presence of good health.

Afterword

I have known Rishma for so many years that calling her just a friend would do injustice to our relationship. She is my family. I have seen her since she was a young girl studying day and night for her medical exams. Every time I visited my friend and her sister Poonam Dhillon those days, I would find Rishma studying! Even then I would tell her that once she becomes a doctor I will definitely come to her because I have seen how hard she has worked to achieve this. So it's natural that she is the official gynaecologist of the Kolhapure family. My two sisters, Shivangi and Tejaswini, and I always go to Rishma for any gynaecological issues. And what may start as a consultation can end up with us spending a long time together, having a blast.

A woman's gynaecologist can become her close friend. After all, you share your innermost thoughts and concerns with her and can discuss any issue privately, knowing that she will not disclose it to anyone. And taking and heeding her good advice can help you remain healthy and fit.

I wish her immense success for this much needed book, *Fit at 40*. I am sure it will guide many women who are confused about problems that they face for the first time in their 40s and are not able to visit a doctor each time. It gives precise information, which is more useful than going through hundreds of pages and conflicting opinions on the Internet.

I am in my mid-40s and Rishma has held my hand through every obstacle this decade had thrown my way. With her, you and I are both in good hands.

Padmini Kolhapure

Notes

1: Physical Changes

1. Cited from an article titled, '5 Steps to Conquering Your Over-40 Belly', http://www.doctoroz.com/videos/5-steps-conquering-your-over-40-belly?hs317=billboard_5
2. Cited from an article titled, 'Revealed: Three quarters of women so embarrassed by "bingo wings" that they've stopped waving', http://www.dailyrecord.co.uk/lifestyle/health-fitness/revealed-three-quarters-of-women-so-embarrassed-1077412
3. Cited from an article titled, 'Hormones And Weight Gain In Women Over 40', http://www.amberen.com/about-menopause/symptoms-of-menopause/hormones-and-weight-gain-in-women-over-40/
4. Cited from an article titled, 'The story of perimenopause symptoms around the world', http://www.natural-

menopause-journey.com/perimenopause-symptoms-and-culture.html

5. Cited from an article titled, 'Osteoporosis and Hip Fracture', http://www.hips-protect.com/osteoporosis
6. Cited from an article in the *Indian Express* titled, 'Osteoporosis can hit the young too, courtesy lifestyle', http://www.indianexpress.com/news/-osteoporosis-can-hit-the-young-too-courtesy-lifestyle-/531280/
7. Cited from an article in the *Optometry Times* titled, 'Women at higher risk for vision impairment', http://optometrytimes.modernmedicine.com/optometrytimes/news/tags/glaucoma/women-higher-risk-vision-impairment
8. Cited from an article in the *Daily Mail* titled, 'Can a sexless marriage be happy?', http://www.dailymail.co.uk/home/you/article-432464/Can-sexless-marriage-happy.html

2: Cognitive Changes

1. Cited from an article in the *Daily Mail* titled, 'The menopause "can cause memory loss": Scientists say fluctuating levels of female hormones are behind the problem', http://www.dailymail.co.uk/health/article-2256675/Does-menopause-really-make-forgetful-Yes-long-say-scientists.html
2. Cited from an article by Vincent T. Martin, MD, Department of Internal Medicine, University of Cincinnati

College of Medicine, Cincinnati Ohio, in an article tilted 'Menstrual Migraine: New Approaches to Diagnosis and Treatment', http://www.americanheadachesociety.org/assets/1/7/Vincent_Martin_-_Menstrual_Martin.pdf

3: Psychological Changes

1. Cited from an article titled, 'Personality changes with age', http://www.webmd.com/mental-health/news/20030512/personality-changes-with-age
2. Cited from an article titled, 'Depression and lifestyle in Indian ageing women', http://medind.nic.in/jak/t09/i1/jakt09i1p73.pdf

4: Bleeding

1. Cited from an article in the *Daily Mail* titled, 'HRT is safe to combat menopause, say experts', http://www.dailymail.co.uk/health/article-2336605/HRT-IS-safe-combat-menopause-say-experts-After-decade-controversy-benefits-thought-outweigh-risks.html

5: Unplanned Pregnancies

1. Cited from an article titled, 'The Potential of Long-acting Reversible Contraception to Decrease Unintended Pregnancy', http://www.arhp.org/publications-and-resources/contraception-journal/september-2008

2. Cited from an article titled, 'But we used a condom,' http://tvtropes.org/pmwiki/pmwiki.php/Main/ButWeUsedACondom

10: Fertility

1. Cited from an article titled, 'Here's how your sick sperm hurts your wife', http://www.chesstango.com/2013/08/heres-how-your-sick-sperm-hurts-your-wife-may-be-due-to-the-fact-that-your-sperm-is-defective-a-must-read/

11: Gynaecological Cancers

1. Cited from an article titled, 'Dogs trained to help sniff out ovarian cancers', http://www.usatoday.com/story/news/nation/2013/08/09/dogs-ovarian-cancer/2635249/

Acknowledgements

This book would not have been possible without the constant support and encouragement of my husband Dr Hrishikesh Pai, my pillar of strength and my lifeline.

My sister Poonam Dhillon who has shaped and moulded me from childhood and made me the person I am. She has been a mother, sister, and best friend to me always.

My children Arnav and Anvisha who have never complained about how busy I am and have grown to become independent and responsible young adults who have made me proud.

My three very distinguished contributors—Dr Purnima Mhatre, Dr Savita Davre, and Leena Mogre– all famous and busy practitioners in their own fields, who immediately agreed to contribute to the book.

Raveena Tandon and Padmini Kolhapure who so kindly wrote the Foreword and Afterword.

My secretary Sonali Nougam who efficiently did all the work associated with the book.

Parita Patel whose inputs at every stage of the book writing were very helpful.

Gurveen, Milee, and everyone at Random House who gave me a free hand and accommodated all my requests.

Last but not the least, all my patients over the years who have had faith in me, loved me, and given me so much warmth and appreciation that it has all been worth it.

A Note on the Author

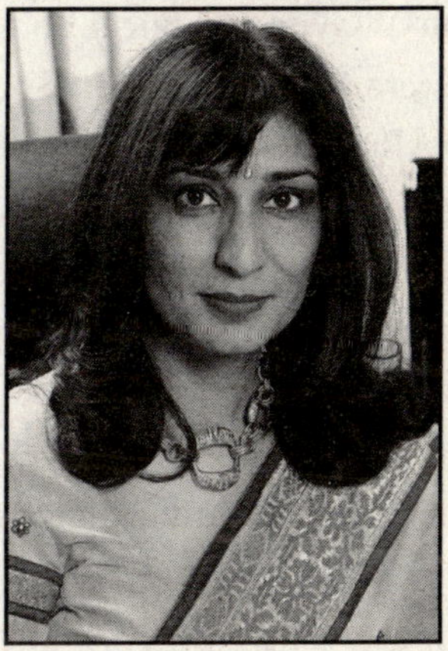

Dr Rishma Dhillon Pai is an honorary consultant gynaecologist at the Jaslok and Lilavati Hospitals, two of the best known hospitals in Mumbai.

Her special interests are infertility, minimal access surgery (keyhole or endoscopic surgery), menopause, and adolescent problems. She has trained in minimal access surgery, IVF, and ICSI at Antwerp, Belgium. She has also trained in egg and embryo freezing at the world's biggest IVF centre in Japan, and also advanced her skills in this field in Italy, China, and Portugal.

Dr Pai has served as the senior vice president of the Federation of Obstetric and Gynaecological Societies of India, which is a large federation of 26,000 gynaecologists of India. She is presently the Jt clinical secretary of MOGS (The Mumbai Obstetric & Gynaecological society), treasurer of Indian Association of Gynaecological Endoscopists (IAGE), and honarary secretary of the Indian Society for Assisted Reproduction (ISAR). She is the first Indian to be elected on the board of the World Endometriosis Society. She was also the chairperson of the Food, Drugs, and Medicosurgical Equipment committee of FOGSI. She was the organizing secretary of the All India Congress of Obstetrics and Gynaecology, AICOG 2013, Mumbai—one of the largest medical conferences in free India attended by more than 10,000 delegates.

Dr Pai is among the first doctors in India to start the procedure of uterine balloon ablation therapy for heavy bleeding. She is one of the first in Asia to offer a non-surgical treatment for the common problem of fibroids, using MRI guided ultrasound. She was one of the first in India to start and teach other gynaecologists the use of abortion pills. She also holds the distinction of having delivered a 60-year-old woman's baby, one of the oldest patients in India. She, along with her husband Dr Hrishikesh Pai, has had the fortune of treating thousands of infertile couples and helped them to have their own child.

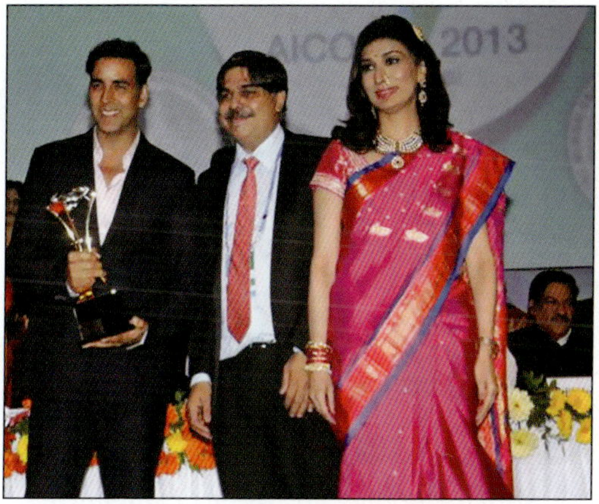

Akshay Kumar, Dr Hrishikesh Pai, and Dr Rishma Dhillon Pai

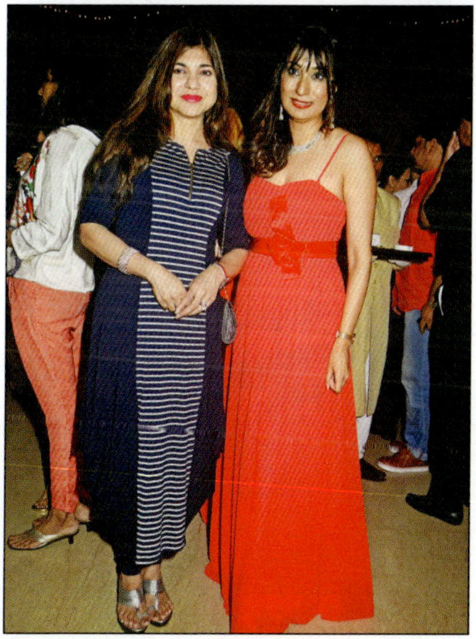

Alka Yagnik and Dr Rishma Dhillon Pai

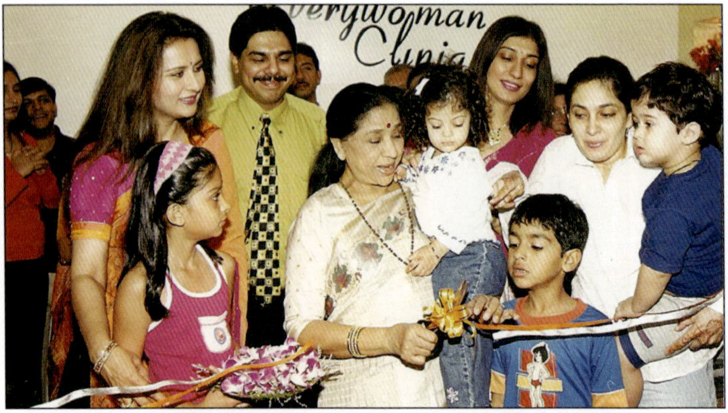

Asha Bhosle inaugurating Dr Rishma Dhillon Pai's clinic

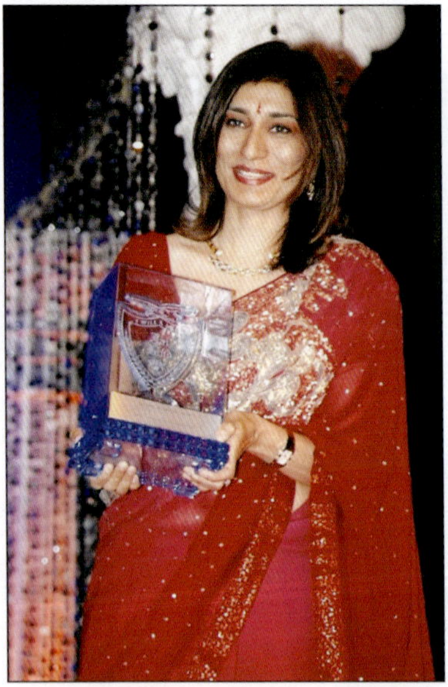

Dr Rishma Dhillon Pai receiving the distinguished alumni award from Jaihind College

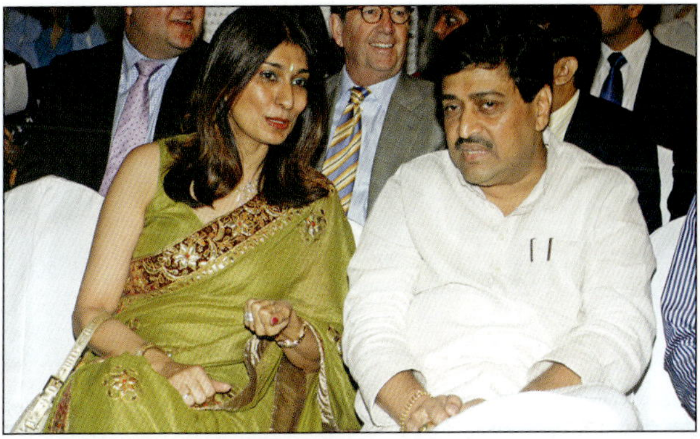

Dr Rishma Dhillon Pai and Shri Ashok Chavan ji (Former Chief Minister of Maharashtra)

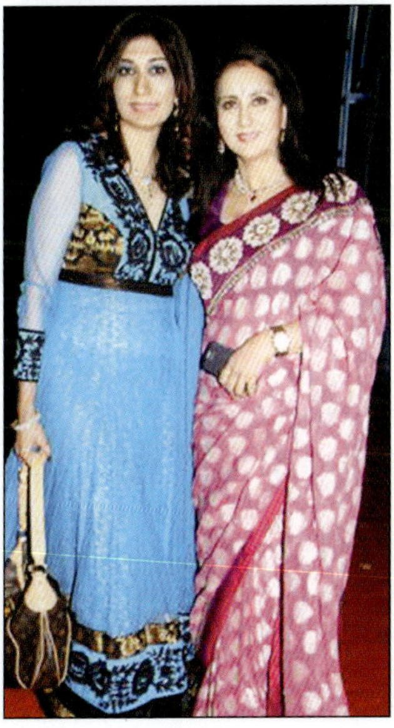

Dr Rishma Dhillon Pai with sister Poonam Dhillon

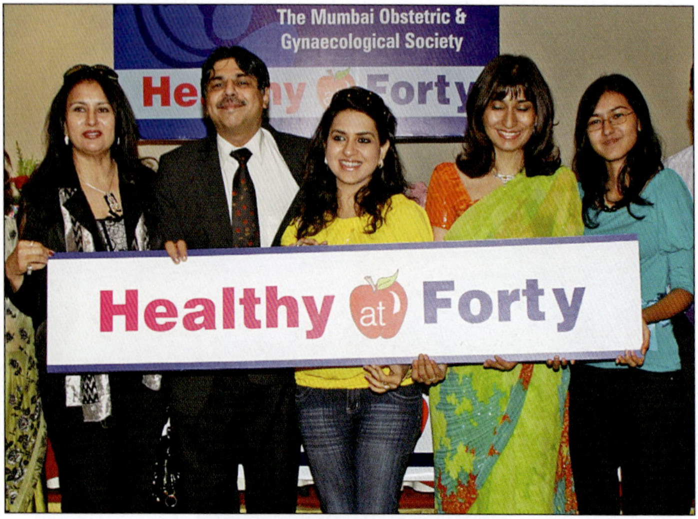

Poonam Dhillon, Dr Hrishikesh Pai, Shaina NC, Dr Rishma Dhillon Pai, and Anvisha Pai

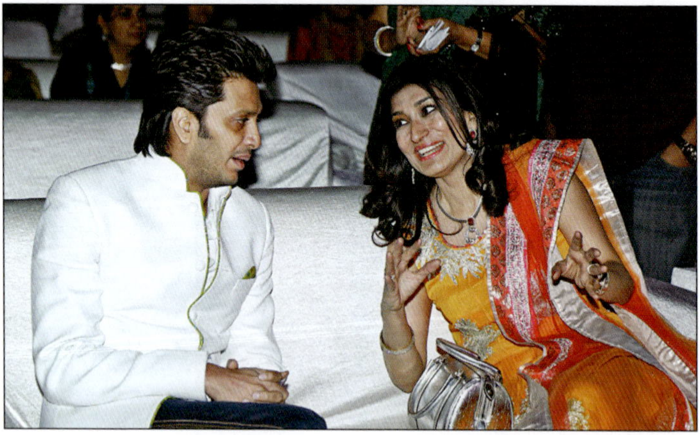

Dr Rishma Dhillon Pai and Ritesh Deshmukh

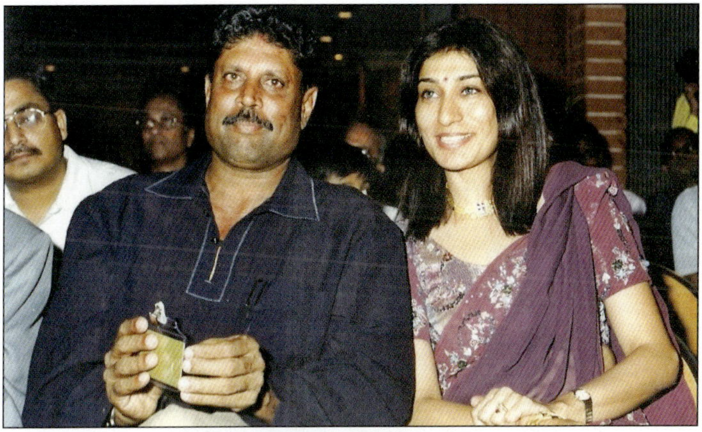

Kapil Dev and Dr Rishma Dhillon Pai

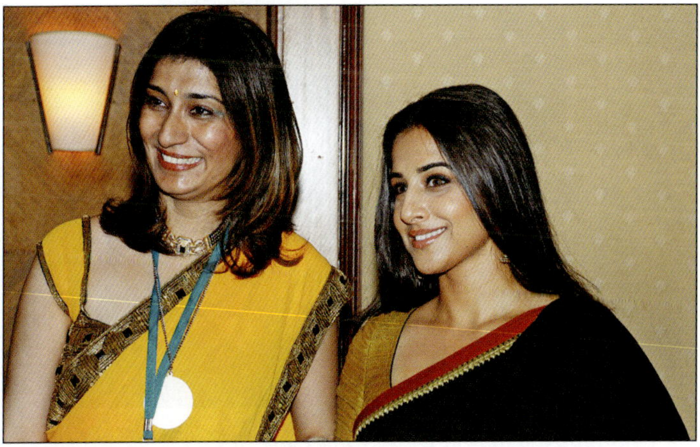

Dr Rishma Dhillon Pai with Vidya Balan

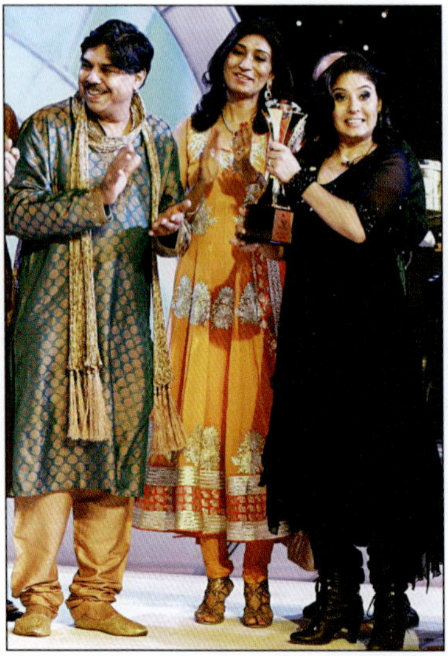

With Dr Hrishikesh Pai and Sunidhi Chauhan

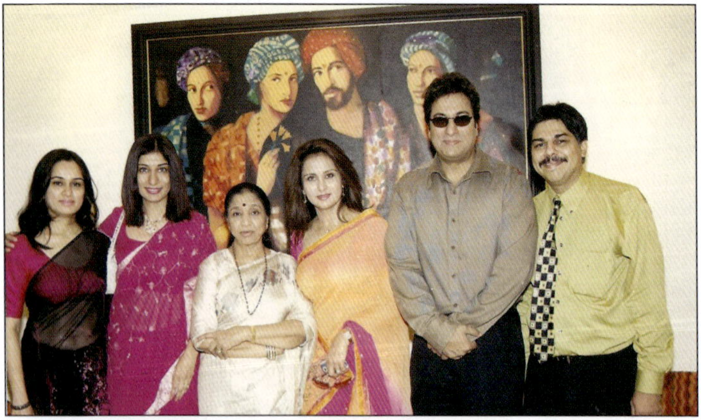

Padmini Kolhapure, Dr Rishma Dhillon Pai, Asha Bhosle, Poonam Dhillon, Talat Aziz, and Hrishikesh Pai

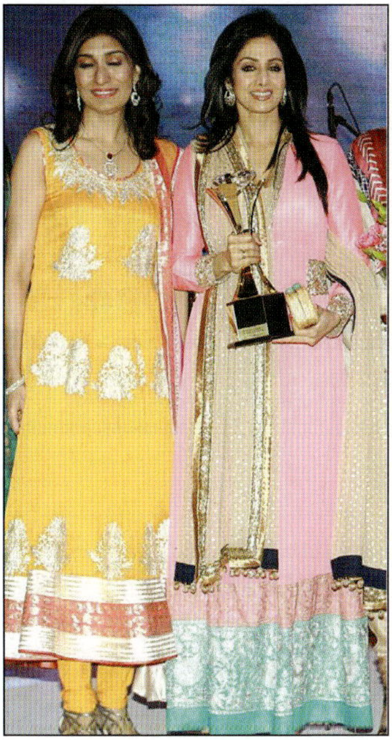

With Sridevi

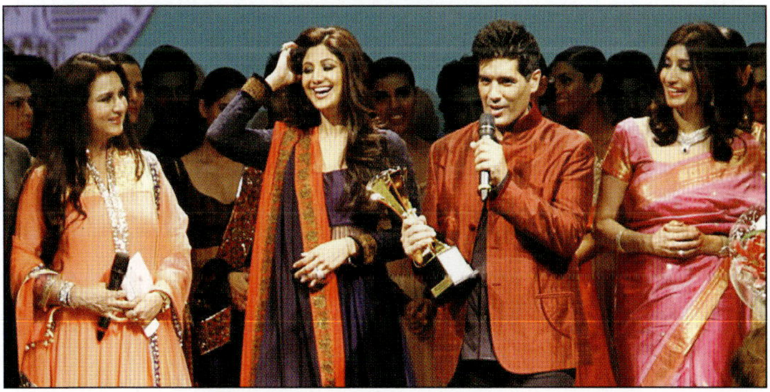

Poonam Dhillon, Shilpa Shetty, Manish Malhotra, and Dr Rishma Dhillon Pai

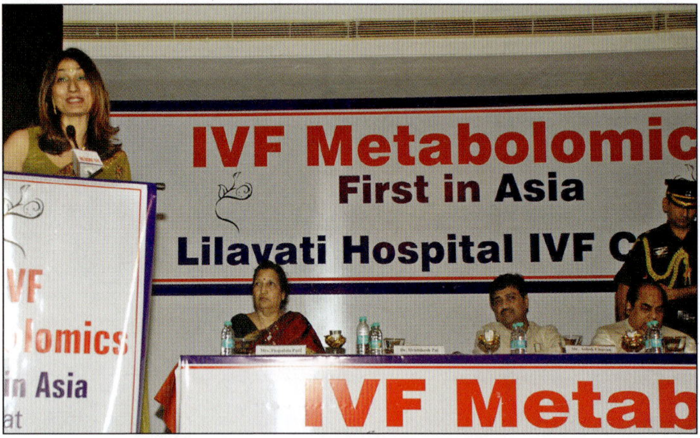

With Mrs Patil, Shri Ashok Chavan ji, and Hon. Governor Dr D. Y. Patil

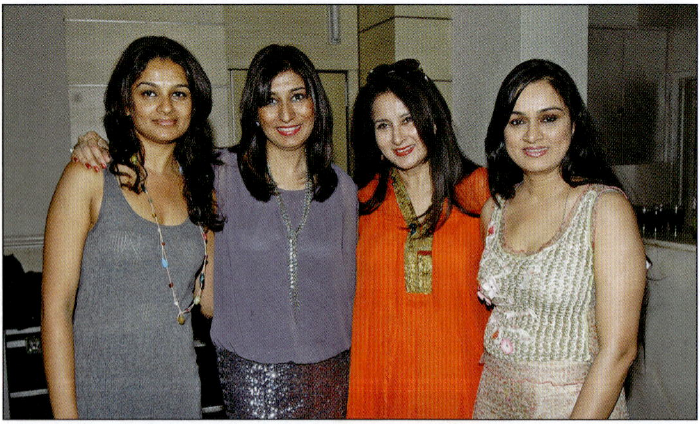

Tejaswini Kolhapure, Dr Rishma Dhillon Pai, Poonam Dhillon, and Padmini Kolhapure